Management of Pancreatic Diseases

Editor

NUZHAT A. AHMAD

GASTROENTEROLOGY CLINICS OF NORTH AMERICA

www.gastro.theclinics.com

Consulting Editor
GARY W. FALK

March 2016 • Volume 45 • Number 1

ELSEVIER

1600 John F. Kennedy Boulevard • Suite 1800 • Philadelphia, Pennsylvania, 19103-2899
http://www.theclinics.com

GASTROENTEROLOGY CLINICS OF NORTH AMERICA Volume 45, Number 1
March 2016 ISSN 0889-8553, ISBN-13: 978-0-323-41647-4

Editor: Kerry Holland
Developmental Editor: Alison Swety

Gastroenterology Clinics of North America (ISSN 0889-8553) is published quarterly by Elsevier Inc., 360 Park Avenue South, New York, NY 10010-1710. Months of issue are March, June, September, and December. Business and Editorial Offices: 1600 John F. Kennedy Blvd., Suite 1800, Philadelphia, PA 19103-2899. Customer Service Office: 6277 Sea Harbor Drive, Orlando, FL 32887-4800. Periodicals postage paid at New York, NY and additional mailing offices. Subscription prices are $320.00 per year (US individuals), $100.00 per year (US students), $587.00 per year (US institutions), $350.00 per year (Canadian individuals), $720.00 per year (Canadian institutions), $445.00 per year (international individuals), $220.00 per year (international students), and $720.00 per year (international institutions). Foreign air speed delivery is included in all *Clinics* subscription prices. All prices are subject to change without notice. **POSTMASTER**: Send address changes to *Gastroenterology Clinics of North America*, Elsevier Health Sciences Division, Subscription Customer Service, 3251 Riverport Lane, Maryland Heights, MO 63043. **Telephone: 1-800-654-2452 (U.S. and Canada); 314-447-8871 (outside U.S. and Canada). Fax: 314-447-8029. E-mail: journalscustomerservice-usa@elsevier.com (for print support);** journalsonlinesupport-usa@elsevier.com (for online support).

Reprints. For copies of 100 or more, of articles in this publication, please contact the Commercial Reprints Department, Elsevier Inc., 360 Park Avenue South, New York, New York 10010-1710. Tel. 212-633-3874, Fax: 212-633-3820, E-mail: reprints@elsevier.com.

Gastroenterology Clinics of North America is also published in Italian by Il Pensiero Scientifico Editore, Rome, Italy; and in Portuguese by Interlivros Edicoes Ltda., Rua Commandante Coelho 1085, 21250 Cordovil, Rio de Janeiro, Brazil.

Gastroenterology Clinics of North America is covered in *MEDLINE/PubMed (Index Medicus), Excerpta Medica, Current Contents/Clinical Medicine, Science Citation Index, ISI/BIOMED,* and *BIOSIS.*

Contributors

CONSULTING EDITOR

GARY W. FALK, MD, MS
Professor of Medicine, Division of Gastroenterology, Hospital of the University of Pennsylvania, University of Pennsylvania Perelman School of Medicine, Philadelphia, Pennsylvania

EDITOR

NUZHAT A. AHMAD, MD, AGAF
Associate Professor, Division of Gastroenterology, Department of Medicine, University of Pennsylvania Perelman School of Medicine, Philadelphia, Pennsylvania

AUTHORS

SUNIL AMIN, MD, MPH
Clinical Fellow, Division of Gastroenterology, Department of Medicine, Icahn School of Medicine at Mount Sinai, New York, New York

VINAY CHANDRASEKHARA, MD
Assistant Professor of Medicine, Division of Gastroenterology, University of Pennsylvania Perelman School of Medicine, Philadelphia, Pennsylvania

JASHODEEP DATTA, MD
Division of Gastrointestinal Surgery, Department of Surgery, University of Pennsylvania Perelman School of Medicine, Philadelphia, Pennsylvania

JAMES J. FARRELL, MD
Director, Yale Center for Pancreatic Disease, Section of Digestive Disease, Yale University, New Haven, Connecticut

TIMOTHY B. GARDNER, MD, MS
Associate Professor, Geisel School of Medicine at Dartmouth, Hanover, New Hampshire; Associate Professor of Medicine, Section of Gastroenterology and Hepatology, Dartmouth Hitchcock Medical Center, Lebanon, New Hampshire

PHILLIP S. GE, MD
Division of Digestive Diseases, David Geffen School of Medicine at UCLA, Los Angeles, California

SHILPA GROVER, MD, MPH
Division of Gastroenterology, Brigham and Women's Hospital, Harvard Medical School, Boston, Massachusetts

KUNAL JAJOO, MD
Division of Gastroenterology, Brigham and Women's Hospital, Harvard Medical School, Boston, Massachusetts

NIGEEN H. JANISCH, MD
Geisel School of Medicine at Dartmouth, Hanover, New Hampshire

GYANPRAKASH A. KETWAROO, MD, MSc
Assistant Professor of Medicine, Division of Gastroenterology, Baylor College of Medicine, Houston, Texas

MICHELLE KANG KIM, MD, PhD
Associate Director of Endoscopy, Division of Gastroenterology, Associate Professor, Department of Medicine, Icahn School of Medicine at Mount Sinai, New York, New York

KAMRAAN MADHANI, MD
Yale-Waterbury Internal Medicine Residency Program, Yale University School of Medicine, New Haven, Connecticut

KOENRAAD J. MORTELE, MD
Associate Professor of Radiology, Harvard Medical School; Division of Abdominal Imaging, Department of Radiology, Beth Israel Deaconess Medical Center, Boston, Massachusetts

ALI NAJI, MD, PhD
Professor, Division of Transplantation, Department of Surgery, University of Pennsylvania Perelman School of Medicine, Philadelphia, Pennsylvania

JON S. ODORICO, MD
Professor, Division of Transplantation, Department of Surgery, University of Wisconsin School of Medicine and Public Health, Madison, Wisconsin

ROBERT R. REDFIELD, MD
Assistant Professor, Division of Transplantation, Department of Surgery, University of Wisconsin School of Medicine and Public Health, Madison, Wisconsin

MICHAEL R. RICKELS, MD, MS
Associate Professor, Division of Endocrinology, Diabetes & Metabolism, Department of Medicine, University of Pennsylvania Perelman School of Medicine, Philadelphia, Pennsylvania

BRIAN P. RIFF, MD
Advanced Endoscopy Fellow, Division of Gastroenterology, Icahn School of Medicine at Mount Sinai, New York, New York

MANDEEP S. SAWHNEY, MD, MS
Assistant Professor of Medicine, Harvard Medical School; Division of Gastroenterology, Beth Israel Deaconess Medical Center, Boston, Massachusetts

AMRITA SETHI, MD
Assistant Professor of Medicine, Division of Digestive and Liver Disease, Columbia University Medical Center, New York, New York

CHARLES M. VOLLMER Jr, MD
Division of Gastrointestinal Surgery, Department of Surgery, University of Pennsylvania Perelman School of Medicine, Philadelphia, Pennsylvania

RABINDRA R. WATSON, MD
Division of Digestive Diseases, David Geffen School of Medicine at UCLA, Los Angeles, California

MIKHAYLA WEIZMANN
Department of Health Sciences, University of Missouri, Columbia, Missouri

MING-MING XU, MD
Fellow in Gastroenterology, Division of Digestive and Liver Disease, Columbia University Medical Center, New York, New York

Contents

This article reviews advances in the management of acute pancreatitis. Medical treatment has been primarily supportive for this diagnosis, and, despite extensive research efforts, there are no pharmacologic therapies that improve prognosis. The current mainstay of management, notwithstanding the ongoing debate regarding the volume, fluid type, and rate of administration, is aggressive intravenous fluid resuscitation. Although antibiotics were used consistently for prophylaxis in severe acute pancreatitis to prevent infection, they are no longer used unless infection is documented. Enteral nutrition, especially in patients with severe acute pancreatitis, is considered a cornerstone in management of this disease.

Endoscopic drainage is the first-line therapy in the management of pancreatic pseudocysts. Before endoscopic drainage, clinicians should exclude the presence of pancreatic cystic neoplasms and avoid drainage of immature peripancreatic fluid collections or pseudoaneurysms. The indication for endoscopic drainage is not dependent on absolute cyst size alone, but on the presence of attributable signs or symptoms. Endoscopic management should be performed as part of a multidisciplinary approach in close cooperation with surgeons and interventional radiologists. Drainage may be performed either via a transpapillary approach or a transmural approach; additionally, endoscopic necrosectomy may be performed for patients with walled-off necrosis.

There is an evolving understanding that autoimmune pancreatitis (AIP) is an immunoglobulin (Ig) G4 systemic disease. It can manifest as primarily a pancreatic disorder or in association with other disorders of presumed autoimmune cause. Classic clinical characteristics include obstructive jaundice, abdominal pain, and acute pancreatitis. Thus, AIP can be difficult to distinguish from pancreatic malignancy. However, AIP may respond to therapy with corticosteroids, and has a strong association with other immune mediated diseases. Although primarily a pathologic diagnosis, attempts have been made to reliably diagnose AIP clinically. AIP can be classified as either type 1 or type 2.

visualize the pancreas in even higher resolution and diagnose premalignant and malignant lesions of the pancreas with improved accuracy. This report reviews the range of imaging tools currently available to evaluate pancreatic lesions, from solid tumors to pancreatic cysts.

Pancreatic adenocarcinoma is a leading cause of cancer death. Few patients are candidates for curative resection due to the late stage at diagnosis. While most pancreatic adenocarcinomas are sporadic, approximately 10% have an underlying hereditary basis. Known genetic syndromes account for only 20% of the familial clustering of pancreatic cancer cases. The majority are due to non-syndromic aggregation of pancreatic cancer cases or familial pancreatic cancer. Screening aims to identify high-risk lesions amenable to surgical resection. However, the optimal interval for screening and the management of pancreatic cancer precursor lesions detected on imaging are controversial.

The surgical management of pancreatic diseases is rapidly evolving, encompassing advances in evidence-driven selection of patients amenable for surgical therapy, preoperative risk stratification, refinements in the technical conduct of pancreatic operations, and quantification of postoperative morbidity. These advances have resulted in dramatic reductions in mortality following pancreatic surgery, particularly at high-volume pancreatic centers. Surgical decision making is complex, and requires an intimate understanding of disease pathobiology, host physiology, technical considerations, and evolving trends. This article highlights key developments in the contemporary surgical management of pancreatic diseases.

The field of pancreas transplantation has evolved from an experimental procedure in the 1980s to become a routine transplant in the modern era. With short- and long-term outcomes continuing to improve and the significant mortality, quality-of-life, and end-organ disease benefits, pancreas transplantation should be offered to more patients. In this article, we review current indications, patient selection, surgical considerations, complications, and outcomes in the modern era of pancreas transplantation.

GASTROENTEROLOGY
CLINICS OF NORTH AMERICA

THE CLINICS ARE AVAILABLE ONLINE!
Access your subscription at:
www.theclinics.com

Preface

Advances in Management of Pancreatic Diseases

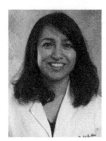

Nuzhat A. Ahmad, MD, AGAF
Editor

"Don't mess with the pancreas" is an old adage oft repeated in hospital corridors and operating theaters. This axiom is a reflection on the fragility as well as the complexity of the pancreas, one of the most fascinating organs in the human body. Management of pancreatic diseases continues to present challenging dilemmas for the clinician. Questions such as "should I start antibiotics on my patient with acute pancreatitis and fever?," "is this patient a candidate for endoscopic drainage of a pseudocyst?," and "what do I do with this 2-cm asymptomatic pancreatic cyst?" are routinely asked in clinical practice. The evolution of our understanding of pancreatic diseases and their management has overall evolved to a more evidence-based approach. Management paradigms continue to shift as more research comes to light. Keeping abreast of these advances is imperative for the physician managing patients with pancreatic diseases.

In this issue of *Gastroenterology Clinics of North America*, the focus is on discussing such advances in topics relevant to both the general gastroenterologist and the clinician with a specific interest in the pancreas. Our authors include a multidisciplinary group of recognized and emerging thought-leaders in their respective fields. A review of this issue will enable the clinician to have a better understanding of the advances in the diagnosis and management of acute pancreatitis, autoimmune pancreatitis, pancreatic cysts, and islet cell tumors of the pancreas. In addition, we have also included articles on screening for pancreatic cancer in the high-risk population—a topic that generates quite a bit of discussion and controversy at conferences. Finally, our surgical colleagues have provided comprehensive and crisp overviews of pancreas transplantation and advances in surgical management of pancreatic diseases.

I am indebted to the team of authors, who have been generous with their time and expertise in writing for this review. I am hopeful that readers will find this issue

Gastroenterol Clin N Am 45 (2016) xi–xii
http://dx.doi.org/10.1016/j.gtc.2015.12.001
0889-8553/16/$ – see front matter © 2016 Published by Elsevier Inc.

gastro.theclinics.com

informative and edifying, with insights that will help them in the management of their patient with pancreatic diseases.

Nuzhat A. Ahmad, MD, AGAF
Division of Gastroenterology
Department of Medicine
Perelman School of Medicine
University of Pennsylvania
PCAM South, 7th Floor
3400 Civic Center Boulevard
Philadelphia, PA 19104, USA

E-mail address:
nuzhat.ahmad@uphs.upenn.edu

Advances in Management of Acute Pancreatitis

Nigeen H. Janisch, MD[a], Timothy B. Gardner, MD, MS[a,b],*

KEYWORDS

- Acute pancreatitis • Medical management • Fluid resuscitation • Antibiotics
- Walled-off pancreatic necrosis • Bedside Index for Severity in Acute Pancreatitis
- Prognostication

KEY POINTS

- Early aggressive fluid resuscitation with lactated Ringer's with a goal total infusion of 2.5 to 4 L in the first 24 hours is recommended.
- Antibiotics are not recommended for prophylaxis of infected pancreatic necrosis although are indicated if another source of infection is clinically suspected.
- Enteral feeding if tolerated is strongly preferred over parenteral feeding, especially in severe acute pancreatitis.
- Endoscopic retrograde cholangiopancreatogrpahy in acute gallstone pancreatitis should not be performed unless there is evidence of ascending cholangitis or there is clinical deterioration in the context of increasing liver test values.
- Cholecystectomy is recommended before discharge for those with acute pancreatitis and gallstones found on imaging.

INTRODUCTION

Acute pancreatitis is a frequently devastating pancreatic inflammation that has been associated with significant morbidity, mortality, and hospitalization costs.[1] The incidence of acute pancreatitis has been increasing and features an overall mortality rate of 5% that may be as high as 30% in the most severe cases.[2–4] It was the most common inpatient gastrointestinal diagnosis in 2009, totaling more than 270,000 United States hospitalizations and incurring costs of more than 2.6 billion dollars.[5] The updated Atlanta classification divides acute pancreatitis into mild and

Disclosures: The authors have no disclosures.
[a] Geisel School of Medicine at Dartmouth, Hanover, NH, USA; [b] Section of Gastroenterology and Hepatology, Dartmouth Hitchcock Medical Center, One Medical Center Drive, Lebanon, NH 03756, USA
* Corresponding author. Section of Gastroenterology and Hepatology, Dartmouth Hitchcock Medical Center, One Medical Center Drive, Lebanon, NH 03756.
E-mail address: timothy.b.gardner@hitchcock.org

severe types.[6,7] Mild, characterized by pancreatic inflammation without necrosis or organ failure, is known as interstitial edematous pancreatitis, which is usually self-limiting and resolves in about 1 week. Severe pancreatitis, occurring in about 20% of cases, predisposes to local complications such as pancreatic necrosis, abscess formation, and pseudocysts. Severe pancreatitis is subdivided further into moderate and severe depending on the presence and duration (>48 hours) of organ failure. This article details treatment of acute pancreatitis, including highlighting new insights into prognostication and focusing on intravenous fluid resuscitation and the current evidence behind the use of antibiotics and pharmacologic therapies.

PREDICTING SEVERITY

- *Simple, universally obtainable markers such as the change in blood urea nitrogen (BUN) level are equally predictive of severity when compared with more complicated systems.*

Predicting the severity of acute pancreatitis can be challenging. Since 1974, when the Ranson's criteria were first proposed, multiple scoring systems (ie, APACHE-II, Bedside Index for Severity in Acute Pancreatitis [BiSAP], Marshall Score) were developed as a means of improving the ability to predict severity in acute pancreatitis. However, despite the use of these often complex systems, laboratory abnormalities in hematocrit, creatinine, and BUN can be used as effective prognostic indicators with equivalent accuracy. For example, an increased risk of pancreatic necrosis has been linked with an elevated hematocrit level at admission or within the first 24 hours as well as an elevated creatinine level within the first 48 hours.[8–10] With regard to BUN, A 2011 meta-analysis of 1043 acute pancreatitis cases found that a BUN $\geq$20 mg/dL (odds ratio, 4.6 and 4.3, respectively) at admission, or an increase in levels within the first 24 hours, was associated with an increased risk of mortality and death.[11] Thus, it is recommended that a simple marker, such as BUN, be used as means of assessing severity and potential progression to organ failure.

FLUID RESUSCITATION

- *The goal is to decrease hematocrit and BUN levels within the first 24 hours of hospitalization.*
- *The goal is early aggressive fluid resuscitation with 250 to 500 mL/h of isotonic crystalloid in the first 12 to 24 hours or urine output of at least 0.5 mL/kg/h.*
- *Lactated Ringer's solution should be used as the resuscitation fluid of choice.*

Now commonly recognized as the primary form of initial management, the importance of adequate fluid resuscitation cannot be understated. In severe cases, acute pancreatitis can lead to pancreatic necrosis and ongoing pancreatic enzyme release.[12] One of the triggers of necrosis is thought to be inadequate glandular perfusion. The pancreatic microcirculation encompasses the celiac and superior mesenteric arteries that branch off to supply the pancreatic acinus. Acute pancreatitis invokes a state of hypovolemia, causing a combination of microangiopathic effects and pancreatic edema that decreases blood flow. This disruption in perfusion may be an important factor responsible for the transition from mild, interstitial edematous disease to severe, necrotizing pancreatitis.[13–17] Current proposed mechanisms of this pathophysiology include hypercoagulability with microthrombi, endothelial damage from free radicals, increased capillary permeability, and hypovolemia.[18] The resultant ischemia produces a flush of cytokines and inflammatory mediators, which can progress into the development of the systemic inflammatory response syndrome (SIRS) and pancreatic necrosis and eventually lead to persistent (>48 hour) organ failure.

As the above data suggest, inadequate fluid resuscitation leading to poor pancreatic microcirculatory perfusion has been associated with acute necrotizing pancreatitis.[19] Specifically, we now know that early fluid resuscitation has more of a therapeutic effect than delayed fluid resuscitation. In one study evaluating specifically the time course of intravenous hydration, early was defined as receiving greater than one-third of the total 72 hours fluid volume within the first 24 hours of hospitalization, whereas late was defined as receiving less than one-third of the total volume.[20] Although the investigation did not focus on the total infused fluid volume, it concluded that the group receiving early fluid resuscitation experienced less mortality than those receiving later resuscitation. Other studies have since supported this claim, including a retrospective analysis of 436 acute pancreatitis patients, which found an association between early fluid resuscitation and decreased SIRS, organ failure at 72 hours, length of hospital stay, and a lower rate of intensive care unit admission.[21]

Although early fluid resuscitation is generally agreed to be an intervention of paramount importance, currently no standard guidelines exist on the optimal fluid type, volume, rate, or duration of treatment.[22] Although human studies regarding the rate of hydration consistently show decreased morbidity and mortality with aggressive hydration in the first 24 hours, the total volume of hydration at the 48-hour mark seems to have a limited effect on patient outcomes. The current American College of Gastroenterology guidelines recommend 250 to 500 mL/h of isotonic crystalloid solution in the first 12 to 24 hours with frequent re-evaluation every 6 hours, with an ultimate goal of decreasing the BUN levels.[23] Some experts recommend that in addition to the 1- to 2-L fluid bolus given in the emergency department, the starting infusion should be at a rate of 250 to 300 mL/h or enough to produce a urine output of at least 0.5 mL/kg/h.[24] The goal within the first 24 hours is a total infusion volume of 2.5 to 4 L, with adjustments to be made based on the patient's age, weight, physical examination, and comorbid conditions.[25]

The type of resuscitation fluid has not been satisfactorily studied. However, in the most widely cited prospective study of fluid resuscitation in acute pancreatitis, Wu and colleagues[26] found that the use of Lactated Ringer's solution, as opposed to normal saline, resulted in less SIRS and a decreased C-reactive protein level at 48 hours. No other prospective fluid studies have evaluated different types of resuscitative fluid, and thus it is generally recommended, in the absence of better evidence, that Lactated Ringer's solution be used as the resuscitative fluid of choice.

It is also important to recognize the consequences of overresuscitation—most notably the development of intra-abdominal compartment syndrome. In a study of patients with predicted severe pancreatitis whose hematocrit level was aggressively lowered at the time of admission, those with aggressive lowering of their hematocrit level had greater morbidity and mortality.[27]

PHARMACOLOGIC STRATEGIES
Antibiotics

- *Antibiotics are not recommended for prophylaxis of infected pancreatic necrosis although are indicated if another source of infection is clinically suspected.*

Infected pancreatic necrosis continues to be the most common cause of death in patients with acute pancreatitis who survive the early phase, accounting for up to 70% of all mortality. Although initially present in about 5% of patients with acute pancreatitis, pancreatic necrosis puts patients at a high risk of pancreatic bed infection, occurring in 50% to 70% of cases.[2,6] Antibiotic prophylaxis and therapy have been a long-contested solution to this problem, with the potential for reduction in the morbidity and mortality associated with severe acute pancreatitis.

Use of antibiotics in previous years as prophylaxis for infected necrosis was recommended and common in practice, supported by early research that showed broad-spectrum antibiotics to decrease the rate of infected pancreatic necrosis.[28] A meta-analysis in 2001, which included randomized, controlled trials, compared antibiotic prophylaxis with no prophylaxis in the setting of acute necrotizing pancreatitis.[29] These investigators found a reduction of 21.2% in sepsis and 12.3% in mortality rate in patients receiving prophylactic antibiotics; however, there was no difference in the incidence of pancreatic infection.

Studies since then have continued to have conflicting results, with a meta-analysis published in 2008, which included the same 3 previously mentioned randomized, controlled trials, finding no difference in the rates of pancreatic infection or mortality between the group receiving antibiotics versus the group receiving placebo.[30] An evaluation of the same trials by a Cochrane review confirmed no difference in mortality but found a significant difference with the use of imipenem alone in terms of preventing infection.[31] Most recently in 2011, an evaluation of 14 randomized, controlled trials totaling 841 patients compared those receiving antibiotics with those receiving placebo. No significant differences were reported in mortality, incidence of infected pancreatic necrosis, nonpancreatic infection, and surgical intervention.[32] There may even be an association with antibiotic use and pancreatic fungal infections.[33]

There has been some consideration of using probiotics for prevention of infection in acute pancreatitis; however, a meta-analysis in 2009 found no reduction in the risk of pancreatic infection or associated mortality.[34] There may be some benefit in selective gut decontamination, which is the process of using oral antibiotics to eradicate enteric gram-negative rods, thus, reducing bacterial translocation from the gastrointestinal tract into the pancreas, but further studies need to be performed.[35]

Ultimately, prophylactic antibiotics are not recommended for use in acute pancreatitis and should not be administered in the first 24 hours after the episode unless there is clinical suspicion for concurrent extrapancreatic infection. Patients may present initially with sepsis, SIRS, or multiorgan failure. Treatment with antibiotics is appropriate if evaluation of the patient, via blood cultures and fine-needle aspirations of pancreatic necrosis, finds infection. However, if there is no obvious source of infection, antibiotics should be discontinued.[23]

Emerging Pharmacologic Therapies

- *No evidence suggests that any of the current targeted therapies provide benefit.*

Extensive research has evaluated pharmacologic agents, such as somatostatin, octreotide, atropine, glucagon, and cimetidine, that specifically reduce pancreatic secretions. Most of the research has had disappointing outcomes. For example, cimetidine, assessed via a meta-analysis of 5 randomized, controlled trials in 2002, has also proven to be no more effective than placebo in decreasing complications or pain.[36,37]

Because acute pancreatitis features autodigestion from proteases, protease inhibitors would theoretically provide benefit. However, studies on gabexate mesilate and aprotinin have not found an improvement in patient outcomes.[28,38] Numerous other attempts at targeted pharmacologic therapy, such as lexipafant (platelet-activating factor antagonist), antioxidants, corticosteroids, nitroglycerin, interleukin-10 or tumor necrosis factor alpha antibodies, have shown no benefit in the treatment of acute pancreatitis and should not be used at this time.[39]

NONPHARMACOLOGIC STRATEGIES
Nutrition

- *Enteral feeding if tolerated is strongly preferred over parenteral feeding.*
- *For mild acute pancreatitis, start enteral feedings within the first week of hospitalization.*
- *For severe acute pancreatitis, start enteral feedings within the first 72 hours of hospitalization.*

In the past, patients with acute pancreatitis were kept "nothing by mouth" — with the intent of providing pancreatic and bowel rest — until pain resolution. The practice did not have any demonstrable benefit, as bowel rest is associated with intestinal mucosal atrophy and increased infectious complications caused by bacterial translocation.[40] Therefore, to maintain gut barrier function, enteral feeding is preferred over parenteral feeding in the management of acute pancreatitis.[41,42]

In mild acute pancreatitis, early initiation of oral intake with a low-fat soft solid diet is often tolerated and is found to be as equally efficacious as tube feedings.[43] Enteral feeding is recommended within 1 week of hospitalization, typically after cessation of nausea and vomiting, discontinuation of parenteral analgesics, reduction in abdominal pain, and return of bowel sounds.[44]

In patients with severe acute pancreatitis, it is recommended to initiate enteral nutrition via nasoenteric tubes within the first 72 hours of hospitalization. A 2012 meta-analysis of 381 patients with severe acute pancreatitis confirms the benefit of enteral versus parenteral feeding. With 2 groups randomly assigned to receive each variation of nutrition, those with enteral feeding benefitted in mortality, infection, organ failure, and had a lower surgical rate.[45] Nasojejunal feeding has long been preferred, although there is evidence that nasogastric feeding has similar clinical efficacy.[46] Although evidence shows a preference toward enteral feeding, if the patient is unable to tolerate it or not meet nutritional goals, parenteral nutrition should be initiated while maintaining a slow rate of enteral feeding.[23]

Management of Underlying Etiology

- *Evaluation for gallstones should be performed with abdominal ultrasound scan in all acute pancreatitis patients*
- *Cholecystectomy is recommended for those with acute pancreatitis and gallstones found on imaging.*
- *Endoscopic retrograde cholangiopancreatogrpahy (ERCP) should not be used in acute pancreatitis unless there is ascending cholangitis or clinical decompensation in the setting of elevated liver tests.*

Identifying and treating the underlying etiology remains the most effective means of preventing a recurrence of acute pancreatitis. The most common cause is gallstones (40%–70%) followed by alcohol use (25%–35%).[47–49] For this reason, an abdominal ultrasound scan is recommended for all those presenting with acute pancreatitis to evaluate for gallstones; if they are present, an elective cholecystectomy is suggested before discharge.[23]

In patients with acute biliary pancreatitis, ERCP should only be used in the context of ascending cholangitis or worsening liver tests with concomitant clinical deterioration.[23,50] In general, therefore, ERCP should be avoided in the management of acute pancreatitis. The role of ERCP in gallstone pancreatitis is discussed in detail elsewhere in this issue.

Recurrence

The recurrence rate of acute pancreatitis is roughly 25% but can be up to 50% in patients whose predisposing factors have not been identified or addressed.[51] As stated above, identifying and treating the underlying etiology is the most important step in preventing recurrence. In the case of a recurrent episode, additional imaging modalities are recommended to evaluate the anatomy of the region and possibly biliary or pancreatic ductal sludge and obstructive calcifications. A computed tomography scan, magnetic resonance cholangiopancreatography, examination, or endoscopic ultrasound scan may be used to visualize the area effectively.[23]

SUMMARY

Although there continues to be high mortality and morbidity associated with acute pancreatitis, treatment remains largely supportive with early aggressive intravenous fluid resuscitation in the first 24 hours used to maintain the pancreatic microcirculation and prevent progression to severe acute pancreatitis, SIRS, multiorgan failure, and pancreatic necrosis. Optimal type, volume, and rate of infusion for the intravenous fluids require further randomized, controlled trials. No pharmacologic therapies are found to be of benefit in reducing the risk of these devastating complications. Furthermore, antibiotics are not recommended for prophylaxis of infected pancreatic necrosis and have shown no benefit in multiple large-scale studies. Identifying and treating the underlying etiology is the best way to prevent recurrence.

REFERENCES

1. Neoptolemos JP, Raraty M, Finch M, et al. Acute pancreatitis: the substantial human and financial costs. Gut 1998;42:886–91.
2. Mann DV, Hershman MJ, Hittinger R, et al. Multicentre audit of death from acute pancreatitis. Br J Surg 1994;81:890–3.
3. Russo MW, Wei JT, Thiny MT, et al. Digestive and liver disease statistics, 2004. Gastroenterology 2004;126:1448–53.
4. Fagenholz PJ, Castillo CF, Harris NS, et al. Increasing United States hospital admissions for acute pancreatitis, 1988-2003. Ann Epidemiol 2007;17:491–7.
5. Peery AF, Dellon ES, Lund J, et al. Burden of gastrointestinal disease in the United States: 2012 update. Gastroenterology 2012;132:1179–87.
6. Appelros S, Lindgren S, Borgström A. Short and long term outcome of severe acute pancreatitis. Eur J Surg 2001;167:281–6.
7. Banks PA, Bollen TL, Dervenis C, et al. Classification of acute pancreatitis 2012: revision of the Atlanta classification and definitions by international consensus. Gut 2013;62:102–11.
8. Baillargeon JD, Orav J, Ramaqopal V, et al. Hemoconcentration as an early risk factor for necrotizing pancreatitis. Am J Gastroenterol 1998;93:2130–4.
9. Brown A, Orav J, Banks PA. Hemoconcentration is an early marker for organ failure and necrotizing pancreatitis. Pancreas 2000;20:367–72.
10. Muddana V, Whitcomb DC, Khalid A, et al. Elevated serum creatinine as a marker of pancreatic necrosis in acute pancreatitis. Am J Gastroenterol 2009;104:164–70.
11. Wu BU, Bakker OJ, Papachristou GI, et al. Blood urea nitrogen in the early assessment of acute pancreatitis. Arch Intern Med 2011;171:669–76.
12. Takeda K, Mikami Y, Fukuyama S, et al. Pancreatic ischemia associated with vasospasm in the early phase of human acute necrotizing pancreatitis. Pancreas 2005;30:40–9.
13. Hotz HG, Foitzik T, Rohweder J, et al. Intestinal microcirculation and gut permeability in acute pancreatitis: early changes and therapeutic implications. J Gastrointest Surg 1998;2:518–25.

14. Banks PA, Freeman ML. Practice guidelines in acute pancreatitis. Am J Gastroenterol 2006;101:2379–400.
15. Knoefel WT, Kollias N, Warshaw AL, et al. Pancreatic microcirculatory changes in experimental pancreatitis of graded severity in the rat. Surgery 1994;116:904–13.
16. Strate T, Mann O, Kleinhans H, et al. Microcirculatory function and tissue damage is improved after therapeutic injection of bovine hemoglobin in severe acute rodent pancreatitis. Pancreas 2005;30:254–9.
17. Bassi D, Kollias N, Fernandez-del Castillo C, et al. Impairment of pancreatic microcirculation correlates with the severity of acute experimental pancreatitis. J Am Coll Surg 1994;179:257–63.
18. Cuthbertson CM, Christophi C. Disturbances of the microcirculation in acute pancreatitis. Br J Surg 2006;93:518–30.
19. Brown A, Baillargeon JD, Hughes MD, et al. Can fluid resuscitation prevent pancreatic necrosis in severe acute pancreatitis? Pancreatology 2002;2:104–7.
20. Gardner TB, Vege SS, Chari ST, et al. Faster rate of initial fluid resuscitation in severe acute pancreatitis diminishes in-hospital mortality. Pancreatology 2009;9: 770–6.
21. Warndorf MG, Kurtzman JT, Bartel MJ, et al. Early fluid resuscitation reduces morbidity among patients with acute pancreatitis. Clin Gastroenterol Hepatol 2011;9:705–9.
22. Nasr JY, Papachristou GI. Early fluid resuscitation in acute pancreatitis: a lot more than just fluids. Clin Gastroenterol Hepatol 2011;9:633–4.
23. Tenner S, Baillie J, DeWitt J, et al. American College of gastroenterology guideline: management of acute pancreatitis. Am J Gastroenterol 2013;108:1400–15.
24. Talukdar R, Vege SS. Early management of severe acute pancreatitis. Curr Gastroenterol Rep 2011;13:123–30.
25. Besselink M, van Santvoort H, Freeman M, et al. IAP/APA evidence-based guidelines for the management of acute pancreatitis. Pancreatology 2013;13:e1–15.
26. Wu BU, Hwang JQ, Gardner TB, et al. Lactated Ringer's solution reduces systemic inflammation compared with saline in patients with acute pancreatitis. Clin Gastroenterol Hepatol 2011;9(8):710–7.
27. Mao EQ, Fei J, Peng YB, et al. Rapid hemodilution is associated with increased sepsis and mortality among patients with severe acute pancreatitis. Chin Med J 2010;123(13):1639–44.
28. Heinrich S, Schäfer M, Rousson V, et al. Evidence-based treatment of acute pancreatitis: a look at established paradigms. Ann Surg 2006;243:154–68.
29. Sharma VK, Howden CW. Prophylactic antibiotic administration reduces sepsis and mortality in acute necrotizing pancreatitis: a meta-analysis. Pancreas 2001; 22:28–31.
30. Bai Y, Gao J, Zou DW, et al. Prophylactic antibiotics cannot reduce infected pancreatic necrosis and mortality in acute necrotizing pancreatitis: evidence from a meta-analysis of randomized controlled trials. Am J Gastroenterol 2008; 103:104–10.
31. Villatoro E, Mulla M, Larvin M. Antibiotic therapy for prophylaxis against infection of pancreatic necrosis in acute pancreatitis. Cochrane Database Syst Rev 2010;(5):CD002941.
32. Wittau M, Mayer B, Scheele J, et al. Systematic review and meta-analysis of antibiotic prophylaxis in severe acute pancreatitis. Scand J Gastroenterol 2011;46: 261–70.
33. Trikudanathan G, Navaneethan U, Vege SS. Intra-abdominal fungal infections complicating acute pancreatitis: a review. Am J Gastroenterol 2011;106:1188–92.

34. Sun S, Yang K, He X, et al. Probiotics in patients with severe acute pancreatitis: a meta-analysis. Langenbecks Arch Surg 2009;394:171–7.
35. Luiten EJ, Hop WC, Lange JF, et al. Controlled clinical trial of selective decontamination for the treatment of severe acute pancreatitis. Ann Surg 1995;222:57–65.
36. Morimoto T, Noguchi Y, Sakai T, et al. Acute pancreatitis and the role of histamine-2 receptor antagonists: a meta-analysis of randomized controlled trials of cimetidine. Eur J Gastroenterol Hepatol 2002;14:679–86.
37. Uhl W, Buchler MW, Malfertheiner P, et al. A randomized, double blind, multicentre trial of octreotide in moderate to severe acute pancreatitis. Gut 1999;45:97–104.
38. Andriulli A, Leandro G, Clemente R, et al. Meta-analysis of somatostatin, octreotide and gabexate mesilate in the therapy of acute pancreatitis. Aliment Pharmacol Ther 1998;12:237–45.
39. Bang UC, Semb S, Nojgaard C, et al. Pharmacological approach to acute pancreatitis. World J Gastroenterol 2008;14:2968–76.
40. Steinberg W, Tenner S. Medical progress: acute pancreatitis. N Engl J Med 1994;330:1198–210.
41. Petrov MS, Kukosh MV, Emelyanov NV. A randomized controlled trial of enteral versus parenteral feeding in patients with predicted severe acute pancreatitis shows a significant reduction in mortality and in infected pancreatic complications with total enteral nutrition. Dig Surg 2006;23:336–45.
42. Gupta R, Patel K, Calder PC, et al. A randomised clinical trial to assess the effect of total enteral and total parenteral nutritional support on metabolic, inflammatory and oxidative markers in patients with predicted severe acute pancreatitis II (APACHE ≥6). Pancreatology 2003;3:406–13.
43. Eckerwall GE, Tingstedt BB, Bergenzaun PE, et al. Immediate oral feeding in patients with acute pancreatitis is safe and may accelerate recovery–a randomized clinical study. Clin Nutr 2007;26:758–63.
44. Jacobson BC, Vandr Vliet MB, Hughes MD, et al. A prospective, randomized trial of clear liquids versus low-fat solid diet as the initial meal in mild acute pancreatitis. Clin Gastroenterol Hepatol 2007;5:946–51.
45. Yi F, Ge L, Zhao J, et al. Meta-analysis: total parenteral nutrition versus total enteral nutrition in predicted severe acute pancreatitis. Intern Med 2012;51:523–30.
46. Eatock FC, Chong P, Menezes N, et al. A randomized study of early nasogastric versus nasojejunal feeding in severe acute pancreatitis. Am J Gastroenterol 2005;100:432–9.
47. Lankisch PG, Assmus C, Lehnick D, et al. Acute pancreatitis: does gender matter? Dig Dis Sci 2001;46:2470–4.
48. Gullo I, Migliori M, Olah A, et al. Acute pancreatitis in five European countries: etiology and mortality. Pancreas 2002;24:223–7.
49. Lowenfels AB, Maisonneuve P, Sullivan T. The changing character of acute pancreatitis: epidemiology, etiology, and prognosis. Curr Gastroenterol Rep 2009;11:97–103.
50. Freeman ML, DiSario JA, Nelson DB, et al. Risk factors for post-ERCP pancreatitis: a prospective, multicenter study. Gastrointest Endosc 2001;54:425–34.
51. Andersson R, Andersson B, Haraldsen P, et al. Incidence, management and recurrence rate of acute pancreatitis. Scand J Gastroenterol 2004;39(9):891–4.

Pancreatic Pseudocysts
Advances in Endoscopic Management

Phillip S. Ge, MD[a], Mikhayla Weizmann[b], Rabindra R. Watson, MD[a],*

KEYWORDS

- Pancreatic pseudocyst • Pseudocyst drainage • Pancreatic stents
- Endoscopic necrosectomy • Endoscopic ultrasonography
- Endoscopic retrograde cholangiopancreatography

KEY POINTS

- Endoscopic management of pseudocysts and walled-off necrosis should be performed as part of a multidisciplinary approach.
- Exclusion of pancreatic cystic neoplasms and pseudoaneurysms is critical before endoscopic drainage procedures.
- Indications for endoscopic drainage of pseudocysts include signs or symptoms attributable to the lesion, as opposed to large cyst size alone.
- The use of covered metal and lumen-apposing metal stents may improve outcomes compared with plastic stents for transmural drainage.
- New dedicated drainage devices and stents have been developed that may facilitate transmural drainage and necrosectomy.

INTRODUCTION

Pseudocysts complicate approximately 10% to 26% of acute pancreatitis and 20% to 40% of chronic pancreatitis cases.[1] The 2012 Revised Atlanta Classification of Acute Pancreatitis defined pancreatic pseudocysts as well-circumscribed, completely encapsulated fluid collections more than 4 weeks old; surrounded by a nonepithelial wall of fibrous or granulation tissue; homogeneous and without a nonliquid component; and arising as a consequence of acute pancreatitis, chronic pancreatitis, or pancreatic trauma with pancreatic ductal disruption.[2] Pseudocysts are a distinct entity from walled-off necrosis, which is a mature, well-circumscribed, completely

Disclosure: The authors have nothing to disclose.
[a] Division of Digestive Diseases, David Geffen School of Medicine at UCLA, 200 UCLA Medical Plaza, Suite 330-33, Los Angeles, CA 90095, USA; [b] Department of Health Sciences, University of Missouri, 510 Lewis Hall, Columbia, MO 65211, USA
* Corresponding author. Division of Digestive Diseases, David Geffen School of Medicine at UCLA, 200 UCLA Medical Plaza, Suite 330-33, Los Angeles, CA 90095.
E-mail address: rwatson@mednet.ucla.edu

Gastroenterol Clin N Am 45 (2016) 9–27
http://dx.doi.org/10.1016/j.gtc.2015.10.003
0889-8553/16/$ – see front matter Published by Elsevier Inc.

gastro.theclinics.com

encapsulated collection of pancreatic or peripancreatic necrosis that occurs more than 4 weeks after the onset of necrotizing pancreatitis.[2]

Endoscopic drainage has emerged as the first-line therapy in the management of pancreatic pseudocysts as well as walled-off necrosis, with significant advantages compared with surgical and percutaneous drainage.[1] Endoscopic pseudocyst drainage was first described by Sahel and colleagues[3] in the late 1980s, using diathermic transmural access into the pseudocyst followed by placement of a naso-cystic tube for irrigation and drainage.[4] The endoscopic management of pancreatic fluid collections has since evolved significantly with the introduction of endosono-graphic guidance,[5] new catheter delivery systems,[6] and indwelling stents, including novel lumen-apposing covered self-expanding metal stents (LAMS).[7] This article dis-cusses the endoscopic management of pancreatic pseudocysts and walled-off necro-sis, including indications for drainage, endoscopic techniques, efficacy, and comparison with percutaneous and surgical drainage.

INDICATIONS FOR DRAINAGE

In general, the indications for pancreatic pseudocyst drainage include persistent pain attributable to the fluid collection, gastric or duodenal obstruction, biliary obstruction, development of pancreatic ascites or pleural effusion, enlarging size on serial imaging, and signs of pseudocyst infection or bleeding (**Box 1**). Pancreatic pseudocysts should not be drained in the absence of suspected infection if the fluid collection is not mature (ie, less than 4–6 weeks old), or the diagnosis remains in question.

An important step before consideration of drainage is the exclusion of other cystic lesions, such as pancreatic cystic neoplasms. Although pseudocysts account for at least 75% of all pancreatic cystic lesions, they can be difficult to distinguish from pancreatic cystic neoplasms, congenital cysts, and retention cysts, especially in those patients without a clear history of pancreatitis.[1] Such lesions often appear morpholog-ically similar to pseudocysts on cross-sectional imaging, and additional evaluation with endoscopic ultrasonography (EUS) and fine-needle aspiration of the cyst fluid may be necessary before endoscopic drainage.[8]

Box 1
Indications for pseudocyst drainage

Persistent abdominal pain attributable to pancreatic pseudocyst

Gastric or duodenal obstruction

Biliary obstruction

Pancreatic ascites

Development of pleural effusions

Enlarging size on serial abdominal imaging

Pseudocyst infection

Pseudocyst bleeding

Exclusion criteria

Pancreatic cystic neoplasms

Acute peripancreatic fluid collections

Acute necrotic collections

Pancreatic pseudocysts and walled-off necrosis should also be differentiated from acute peripancreatic fluid collections and acute necrotic collections, both of which occur in the acute phase of pancreatitis or necrotizing pancreatitis. These collections have yet to develop an encapsulated, well-defined wall surrounding the fluid collection, and often resolve with expectant management.[2]

Historically, guidelines have mandated drainage if pseudocysts are present for longer than 6 weeks. This recommendation originated from observational studies of the natural history of pancreatic pseudocysts and complications associated with conservative management. Between 1971 and 1976, Bradley and colleagues[9] followed 54 patients with pancreatic pseudocysts by serial clinical and sonographic examination until either spontaneous resolution, development of complications, or loss to follow-up. During the observation period, 41% of patients developed complications including rupture, abscess, jaundice, and hemorrhage, and 20% developed spontaneous cyst resolution. The investigators surmised that prolonged observation of pancreatic pseudocysts past 7 weeks resulted in risks that exceeded those of elective surgery. In contrast, more recent studies have suggested that longer periods of observation are safe and effective in permitting spontaneous resolution in up to 86% of patients over an average 1-year follow-up, with a 3% to 9% rate of serious complications.[10–12]

The decision to pursue pseudocyst drainage should not be based on cyst size alone. Although data regarding pseudocyst size and outcomes have been mixed, a cyst of less than 4 cm has been found to be a predictor of spontaneous resolution.[13–15] In the past, drainage has been indicated for pseudocysts larger than 6 cm because of lower rates of spontaneous resolution and greater risks of complications. A study from Yeo and colleagues[11] of 36 patients with asymptomatic pseudocysts showed that 67% of pseudocysts greater than 6 cm in diameter required surgical treatment, compared with 40% of pseudocysts less than 6 cm in diameter. In contrast, Cheruvu and colleagues[12] showed that the median pseudocyst size of those patients requiring intervention was similar to that of patients who were successfully managed conservatively (8 cm vs 7 cm). Similarly, Nguyen and colleagues[16] determined that a cyst size greater than or less than 6 cm had no effect on rates of spontaneous resolution, need for operative management, complications, cyst recurrence, or mortality. This heterogeneity in data regarding cyst size highlights the primacy of symptoms and regional complications attributable to the cyst when considering cyst drainage.

SURGICAL DRAINAGE

An overview of pancreatic pseudocyst drainage techniques is given in **Box 2**. The surgical management of pancreatic pseudocysts depends on the extent of disease and local expertise, and may include cystenterostomy, partial pancreatic resections, and combined laparoscopic and endoscopic interventions. Laparoscopic surgery, such as laparoscopic anterior transgastric cystogastrostomy and lesser sac posterior cystogastrostomy, results in lower morbidity compared with conventional open surgery.[17,18] Surgical series of patients undergoing laparoscopic pseudocyst drainage have shown success in 95% of cases, with 1% mortality, a 12% complication rate, and 10% conversion rate to open surgery.[17] A study comparing the outcomes of 83 patients who underwent cystogastrostomy by either open, laparoscopic, or endoscopic approaches found comparable overall success rates of more than 90% with open and laparoscopic approaches, with no difference in complication rates.[19]

Box 2
Techniques for pseudocyst drainage

Surgical

Open surgical drainage

Laparoscopic surgical drainage
  Anterior transgastric cystogastrostomy
  Lesser sac posterior cystogastrostomy

Percutaneous

Percutaneous irrigation or drainage

Endoscopic

Single or multiple transmural entry (EUS or non-EUS guided) with nasocystic irrigation

Single entry with percutaneous endoscopic gastrostomy for irrigation

Single or multiple transmural entry with plastic or metal stent placement

Transmural entry with endoscopic necrosectomy

Hybrid

Percutaneous irrigation and endoscopic transmural entry

Percutaneous endoscopic direct necrosectomy

PERCUTANEOUS DRAINAGE

Percutaneous drainage of pancreatic pseudocysts and other peripancreatic fluid collections involves placement of a needle and drainage catheter under ultrasonography or computed tomography (CT) guidance. Following successful drainage of the fluid collection, drainage catheters are kept in place until the daily flow decreases to 5 to 10 mL, with repeat CT imaging confirming resolution of the pseudocyst with the catheter tip remaining within the pseudocyst cavity. At present, percutaneous drainage is preferred for collections that are not adjacent to the gastrointestinal lumen or do not communicate with the pancreatic duct, in patients who have immature infected pseudocysts, or in patients who are poor surgical candidates.[1] Hybrid endoscopic and percutaneous approaches for pancreatic pseudocyst irrigation as well as pancreatic necrosectomy have been described and can be performed in specialized centers under close cooperation between the endoscopist and the interventional radiologist.[20]

ENDOSCOPIC DRAINAGE

Endoscopic drainage has emerged as the first-line therapy in the management of pancreatic pseudocysts.[21–23] Compared with surgical and percutaneous drainage, there are multiple advantages to endoscopic drainage, including the ability to place multiple drains, cystic cavity irrigation via nasocystic tubes, and direct endoscopic necrosectomy, all of which are performed via a minimally invasive approach. In addition, ongoing pancreatic duct disruption, leak, or obstruction may be treated via endoscopic retrograde cholangiopancreatography (ERCP) in a single session[1] (**Fig. 1**). A further advantage is that the development of an enterocystic fistula may reduce the risk of pseudocyst recurrence by allowing pancreatic drainage in cases of disconnected tail syndrome.[24] In addition, endoscopic drainage has been shown to be equally if not more effective than surgical and percutaneous drainage, with lower morbidity and complication rates, particularly with respect to persistent cutaneous

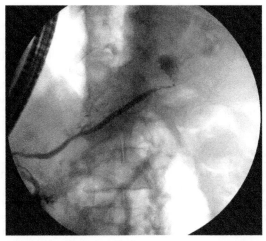

Fig. 1. Pancreatogram showing leak at tail of pancreas.

fistula formation.[21,25] An overview of endoscopic pancreatic pseudocyst drainage techniques is given in **Box 3**. Endoscopic cystogastrostomy, regardless of the technique used, is performed with fluoroscopic guidance.

Transpapillary Drainage

Endoscopic drainage can be performed using either a transpapillary or transmural technique. Endoscopic transpapillary drainage with placement of a pancreatic duct stent is typically reserved for pseudocysts smaller than 6 cm and with communication

Box 3
Endoscopic techniques for pseudocyst drainage
Cyst entry
Transpapillary
Diathermic
Seldinger
EUS Guidance
Single-step access device (Navix system)
Cyst dilation
Balloon dilation
Bougie dilation
Stent placement
Double-pigtail plastic stent
Fully covered self-expanding metal stent (SEMS)
Combination double-pigtail plastic stent within fully covered SEMS
Biflanged covered SEMS (Nagi stent)
Lumen-apposing covered SEMS (Niti-S Spaxus and Axios stents)

to the main pancreatic duct.[26,27] Alternatively, transpapillary stenting is indicated when transmural drainage is not feasible because of contraindications such as coagulopathy, or when the pseudocyst is too distant (>1 cm) from the gastrointestinal lumen to allow safe transmural drainage. Transpapillary stenting may be combined with additional interventions such as major or minor papillotomy, dilation of pancreatic duct strictures, and placement of large-bore pancreatic duct stents across a ductal disruption or into the pseudocyst cavity, if necessary. A combined transmural and transpapillary approach is not typically required for successful resolution of most pancreatic pseudocysts.

Transmural Drainage Without Endoscopic Ultrasound Guidance

Non–EUS-guided transmural drainage requires close proximity of the pseudocyst to the gastrointestinal lumen, as well as endoscopic localization in the form of a visible luminal bulge (**Fig. 2**). There are currently 2 well-described methods for non–EUS-guided cyst entry, known as diathermic puncture and the Seldinger technique.[28,29] Both methods rely on endoscopic needle localization of the point of maximal gastric bulge to confirm the most appropriate location before cystogastrostomy tract dilation and stent placement.

Cyst entry using diathermic puncture involves the use of a needle knife or Cystotome to gain access into and maintain close apposition of the pseudocyst to the gut lumen. The needle knife is directed perpendicularly to the axis of maximal endoscopic bulge. A pure cutting current is then used to gain access into the pseudocyst, with electrocautery discontinued immediately on entry into the cyst cavity to avoid thermal injury to surrounding structures. Once a site is found with suitable fluid return, a small quantity of contrast is injected under fluoroscopic guidance to confirm position within the pseudocyst. Stroking of the needle knife should be avoided, because a cut of even a few millimeters can result in entry of the needle knife into an adjacent gastric vessel. In addition, the needle knife should not extrude consistently in the coaxial plane of cyst entry, because it can result in iatrogenic injury. If blood return is seen once the cyst is punctured, the clinician should immediately consider evaluating for the presence of a pseudoaneurysm or gastric varices.

The Seldinger technique involves creating an initial puncture with an 18-gauge or 19-gauge needle, followed by the introduction of a 0.89-mm (0.035-inch) guidewire

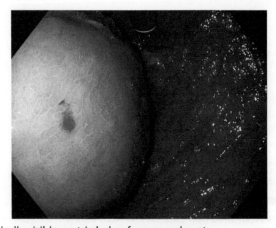

Fig. 2. Endoscopically visible gastric bulge from pseudocyst.

through the needle. In a study of 94 patients, the Seldinger technique was shown to have a comparable efficacy to diathermic puncture (95% vs 92%), although with a significantly lower bleeding complication rate (4.6% vs 15.7%).[29]

Once access into the cyst is obtained with a guidewire, it is looped within the cavity to create 2 to 3 coils, and the needle or catheter is exchanged for a dilating balloon (typically 4-mm, 6-mm, 8-mm, or 10 mm balloons).[1] Inflation of the balloon is then performed under fluoroscopic guidance, with the goal of obliteration of the waist of the balloon, to ensure adequate cystogastrostomy tract dilation. Passage of dilation catheters, such as a 6-French to 10-French bougie, can also be used for tract creation without electrocautery, although cautery access is often still required in cases in which there is minimal endoscopic bulge. Following tract creation and dilation, stents may then be placed for pseudocyst drainage.

Endoscopic Ultrasonography–guided Transmural Drainage

EUS is increasingly used to guide transmural drainage. EUS can be used to exclude pancreatic cystic neoplasms and pseudoaneurysms, and provides real-time image guidance to identify relative contraindications to endoscopic drainage such as gastric varices, cyst-lumen distance greater than 1 cm, and normal intervening pancreatic parenchyma.[30,31] A single-step EUS-guided approach is the most commonly used method for pancreatic pseudocyst drainage.[32] The EUS-guided method involves endosonographically guided puncture of the pseudocyst with a 19-gauge fine-needle aspiration needle. Subsequently, the stylet is withdrawn, cyst aspiration and contrast injection is performed, and a 0.89-mm (0.035-inch) guidewire is placed through the needle for tract dilatation and stent placement (**Fig. 3**).

More recently, a single-step exchange-free access device (Navix; Xlumena, Mountain View, CA) was developed for transluminal pseudocyst drainage.[6] This device comprises an endoscopic trocar with a blade that creates a 3.5-mm puncture

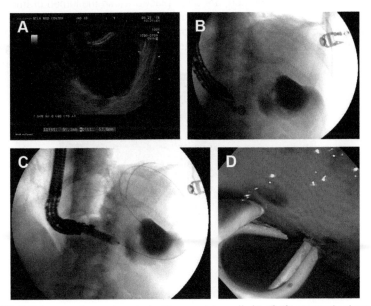

Fig. 3. (*A*) EUS image of pseudocyst abutting gastric wall. (*B, C*) Fluoroscopic views of cyst puncture, contrast injection, wire placement, and dilatation. (*D*) Stent placement.

opening, an anchor balloon that maintains access within the target, a dilation balloon that expands the tract to 10 mm, and 2 guidewire ports for subsequent stent placement. Following EUS-guided transmural entry into the pseudocyst with the trocar, the balloon catheter is then advanced over the trocar, followed by inflation of the anchor balloon. A 0.89-mm (0.035-inch) guidewire is then inserted into the cyst cavity, and the tract is dilated to 10 mm with the dilation balloon. After dilation, a second 0.89-mm (0.035-inch) guidewire is inserted. The access device is then removed from the endoscope, and a 7-French followed by 10-French double-pigtail stent can be inserted in sequence across the guidewire and into the cystogastrostomy tract for drainage. The size of the working channel of current endoscopes limits the first stent to 7-French diameter. Other methods for 1-step simultaneous double-wire pancreatic pseudocyst drainage have also been described.[33,34]

Stent Placement

A variety of different stents are available for pancreatic pseudocyst drainage, including plastic pigtail stents, covered self-expanding metal stents (SEMS), and new LAMS. Based on the currently available literature, the standard of practice in endoscopic drainage of pancreatic pseudocysts remains the placement of multiple double-pigtail plastic stents, with or without a fully covered SEMS.

Transmural pancreatic pseudocyst drainage with plastic stents was first described in 1998,[35] and covered SEMS were introduced in 2010 for transmural necrosectomy.[36] Plastic stents have disadvantages, including a small lumen diameter, which may result in stent occlusion and need for reintervention, hence typically multiple plastic stents are placed in tandem.[37]

SEMS have a much larger luminal diameter than plastic stents and therefore may facilitate greater drainage. However stent migration and tissue injury from stent erosion into either the wall of the pseudocyst or gastrointestinal tract are significant potential adverse events.[38] To prevent migration, double-pigtail plastic stents, ranging in size from 7 French to 10 French, are often placed within the lumen of the covered SEMS to act as an anchor and prevent migration[39] (**Fig. 4**).

Sharaiha and colleagues[40] recently compared metal versus plastic stents for pseudocyst drainage in a retrospective cohort study involving 230 patients who underwent

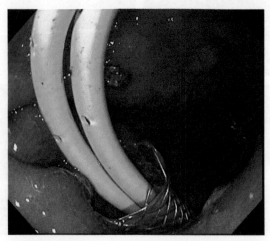

Fig. 4. Fully covered self-expandable metal stent with indwelling anchoring double-pigtail stents.

EUS-guided transmural drainage. They included 118 patients who were drained with double-pigtail plastic stents and 112 patients who were drained using fully covered SEMS. At 12 months, the rate of complete resolution of pseudocysts was significantly lower in the group using double-pigtail plastic stents compared with fully covered SEMS (89% vs 98%; $P = .01$). Procedural adverse events were significantly more common (31% vs 16%; $P = .006$) in the plastic stent group. On multivariate analysis, patients drained with double-pigtail plastic stents were 2.9 times more likely to experience adverse events. The investigators concluded that fully covered SEMS improved clinical outcomes and lowered adverse event rates compared with double-pigtail plastic stents.

A novel metal stent designed for pseudocyst drainage uses round flared ends that may prevent stent migration and tissue injury (Nagi stent, Taewoong Medical Co, Ilsan, South Korea).[41,42] The Nagi stent was recently evaluated by Dhir and colleagues[43] in a prospective single-center study of 47 patients with symptomatic pancreatic pseudocysts in the body and tail of the pancreas. Technical and clinical success was achieved in 43 patients, with 2 patients developing cyst infections. The stent was removed after 3 weeks, at which time patients with a disconnected duct underwent successful ERCP with pancreatic duct stenting. Multivariate analysis suggested that a disconnected duct was an independent predictor of failure at 3 weeks. The investigators concluded that short-term placement of fully covered SEMS with removal after 3 weeks combined with selective pancreatic duct stenting seemed to be safe and effective in the treatment of pseudocysts in the body and tail of the pancreas.

Recently, a second LAMS (Axios; Xlumena, Mountain View, CA) has been developed for use in EUS-guided transmural drainage of pancreatic pseudocysts.[7,44–46] The Axios stent is a nitinol stent that is barbell shaped, flexible, fully covered, and self-expanding (**Fig. 5**). The stent is housed within a catheter-based delivery system and currently is available in 2 sizes: 10-mm and 15-mm diameter by 10-mm length. The 10-mm saddle length is designed to appose the gut lumen to the wall of the pancreatic fluid collection. The large luminal diameter of the stent allows for efficient

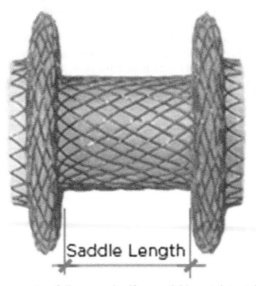

Fig. 5. Axios lumen-apposing, fully covered, self-expandable metal stent. (Image provided courtesy of Boston Scientific. © 2016 Boston Scientific Corporation or its affiliates. All rights reserved.)

drainage of pancreatic pseudocysts, as well as for management of pseudocysts containing necrotic material, including debridement, irrigation, cystoscopy, and necrosectomy. Following resolution of the pancreatic fluid collection, the stent can be removed using a standard endoscopic snare.

The Axios stent was initially evaluated, in a retrospective clinical series, by Itoi and colleagues.[45] They evaluated 15 patients with symptomatic pancreatic pseudocysts, of whom 12 underwent transgastric and 3 underwent transduodenal pseudocyst drainage. Stent placement in 4 of the patients facilitated subsequent endoscopic necrosectomy. All stents were deployed without complication, and all pseudocysts resolved after a single drainage procedure. One stent migrated into the stomach after 19 days, and the remaining 14 stents remained patent at time of removal, with no pseudocyst recurrence over a median follow-up of 11.4 months. The stent was further evaluated in a European retrospective clinical series of 9 patients.[46] All patients achieved complete cyst resolution, device failure occurred in 1 patient, and 1 patient developed cyst recurrence after stent removal. No stent migrations were reported, although 1 patient underwent transesophageal stent placement and developed a tension pneumothorax.

Subsequent larger studies have corroborated the findings of these pilot series using the Axios stent. A large recent European prospective study from Walter and colleagues[47] of 61 patients with pancreatic fluid collections included 46 patients with walled-off necrosis and 15 patients with pancreatic pseudocysts. Technical success was achieved in 98% of patients, and clinical success (defined as resolution of clinical symptoms and decrease in pancreatic fluid collection size <2 cm on imaging) was achieved in 93% of patients with pancreatic pseudocyst and 81% of patients with walled-off necrosis. Treatment failure occurred in 9 patients (16%), 4 of whom required surgical intervention. Stent migration occurred in 3 patients and stent dislodgment during necrosectomy occurred in 3 patients. A total of 5 major complications were reported (9%), including 4 patients with infection of the pancreatic fluid collection and 1 perforation.

A second recent prospective study by Shah and colleagues[7] evaluated the outcomes of Axios stent placement in 33 patients with symptomatic pancreatic pseudocysts and walled-off necrosis, across 7 participating tertiary care centers. The LAMS was placed successfully in 91% of the patients, with 93% resolution of pancreatic fluid collections. Endoscopic debridement across the LAMS was performed in 11 patients. Complications included 3 patients with abdominal pain, 1 patient with stent migration and back pain, and 1 patient with access-site infection and stent dislodgement. The results of this study suggested several advantages of LAMS placement, including single-step deployment, the ability to perform endoscopic debridement with minimal stent migration, and high technical and clinical success rates of greater than 90%.

A similar LAMS (Niti-S Spaxus; Taewoong Medical Co, Ilsan, South Korea) has also been studied in a small retrospective series of 7 patients by Moon and colleagues.[48] The Niti-S Spaxus stent has a flange of 25-mm diameter, and is currently available in 3 sizes: 8-mm, 10-mm, and 16-mm diameter by 5-mm length. Further prospective studies of LAMS are warranted, particularly to elucidate whether the safety and efficacy of LAMS are superior to those of conventional double-pigtail plastic stent placement for pseudocyst drainage.

Walled-off Necrosis

Minimally invasive necrosectomy with endoscopic, percutaneous, and laparoscopic approaches, alone or in combination, have largely replaced traditional open surgical debridement. However, there remains little consensus on the optimal timing and approach. Residual pancreatic necrosis seems to be the most important factor influencing poor endoscopic treatment outcome.[49] Therefore, if necrotic debris is identified during EUS or thick cyst aspirate is encountered during pseudocyst drainage, consideration should be given to placement of larger-bore stents and/or nasocystic tubes for irrigation and drainage. Nasocystic tubes are flushed continuously or lavaged every 3 to 4 hours for several days to weeks depending on the amount of debris present and patient tolerance.[1] If longer-term irrigation is necessary, a percutaneous endoscopic gastrostomy with a catheter placed directly into the cyst fossa is a reasonable alternative.[20]

Endoscopic necrosectomy involves a combination of pseudocyst lavage and mechanical debridement. Direct endoscopic necrosectomy does not need to occur at the time of the index drainage procedure, and may increase the risk of dehiscence between the pseudocyst and the gut lumen. In general, debridement and necrosectomy should be performed through a mature tract, typically a minimum of 2 to 4 weeks after initial cystogastrostomy, although direct debridement following LAMS placement has been described.[1]

Multiple techniques for endoscopic necrosectomy have been reported.[50,51] Conventionally, dilation of the cystogastrostomy tract is performed anywhere from 12 to 20 mm using balloon dilators, to allow for the passage of diagnostic or therapeutic channel gastroscopes into the cavity for debridement. Subsequently, necrosectomy is performed using a combination of snares, graspers, ERCP baskets, and polyp retrieval devices, followed by upsizing of the stents to progressively increase the diameter of the cystogastrostomy (**Fig. 6**). The advent of large-diameter LAMS may more readily facilitate endoscopic debridement and necrosectomy without the need for multiple endoscopic dilations.[7]

Endoscopic necrosectomy is often tedious, time consuming, and labor intensive.[20,52] However, a high success rate has been reported among selected patients. In a multicenter series of 104 patients, Gardner and colleagues[53] reported a success rate of 91%, with a mean time to resolution of 4.1 months. Similarly, in a series of 25 patients, Voermans and colleagues[54] reported a direct endoscopic necrosectomy success rate of 93% with no mortality.

In conjunction with interventional radiology, several hybrid approaches have also been described. Navarrete and colleagues[55] as well as Baron and Kozarek[20] have described collaborative approaches in which a large-bore SEMS is placed percutaneously to allow access for direct endoscopic necrosectomy with a flexible endoscope. This approach allows endoscopic access to areas that are not available from a transluminal approach.[20,55]

Alternatively, Gluck and colleagues[56] described a dual-modality technique with CT-guided percutaneous irrigation/drainage catheter placement combined with internal transmural drainage, which resulted in decreased length of hospitalization and number of radiological and endoscopic procedures compared with either modality alone.[57] Long-term follow-up data of 117 patients who underwent dual-modality drainage over a median duration of 749.5 days showed that this method of treatment results in favorable clinical outcomes, with complete avoidance of pancreaticocutaneous fistulae, surgical necrosectomy, and major procedure-related adverse events, while maintaining a low (3.4%) disease-related mortality.[58]

For complex organized necrosis, Varadarajulu and colleagues[59] described an EUS-guided multiple transluminal gateway technique. The technique involves creating 2 or more transluminal drainage sites to permit irrigation and drainage. First, a cystogastrostomy is performed, followed by balloon dilation to 8 mm and placement of a 7-French double-pigtail stent. Next, EUS guidance is used to locate a second

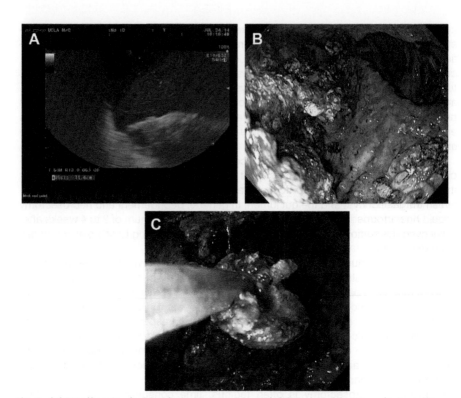

Fig. 6. (*A*) EUS showing hyperechoic necrotic material. (*B*) Endoscopic view of intracystic necrosis. (*C*) Endoscopic necrosectomy.

drainage site distant from the initial site. A cystogastrostomy is then created at the second site, followed by balloon dilation to 15 mm and placement of multiple (2–4) 7-French double-pigtail stents. Subsequently, a 7-French nasocystic drainage catheter is placed into the first site adjacent to the double-pigtail stent. The first site is dilated to only 8 mm to facilitate localization of the second site, because rapid evacuation of pancreatic fluid may preclude such localization. In select patients with very large walled-off pancreatic necrosis, greater than 15 cm in diameter, a third transmural tract can be created with placement of 2 to 4 additional double-pigtail stents. Following the procedure, 200 mL of saline is irrigated every 4 hours through the nasocystic tube, shifting patient position between flushes. Usage of this technique resulted in successful resolution in 11 of 12 (91.7%) patients with symptomatic walled-off pancreatic necrosis, and only 1 patient required endoscopic necrosectomy. In contrast, there was successful resolution in only 25 of 48 (52.1%) patients managed with conventional endoscopic drainage, with 17 patients requiring surgery, 3 patients requiring endoscopic necrosectomy, and 3 patients dying of multiorgan failure.[59]

CLINICAL OUTCOMES OF ENDOSCOPIC DRAINAGE OF PANCREATIC PSEUDOCYSTS

Overall, endoscopic drainage is an excellent first-line therapy for the drainage of pancreatic pseudocysts, with complete resolution of pseudocysts in 71% to 95% of cases, complication rates of 0% to 37%, and procedure-related mortality of 0% to 1%.[6,21–23,26,27,37,44,60–65] However, the various drainage techniques have differed in reported complication and reintervention rates.

In a study by Hookey and colleagues[60] of 116 patients who underwent endoscopic drainage of pancreatic fluid collections by either transmural stenting alone, transpapillary stenting alone, or combined transmural and transpapillary stenting, there was no difference in efficacy between the three methods. However, the complication rates were higher in the transmural and combined groups (10% and 17%, respectively), and the recurrence rate was higher in the combined group compared with either transpapillary or transmural drainage alone. The investigators suggested that the higher recurrence rate in the combined group may be caused by lack of maturation of a transenteric fistula in the setting of transpapillary stenting.

EUS guidance provides real-time image guidance during endoscopic drainage, and thus may improve adverse event rates. Antillon and colleagues[32] reported that single-step EUS guidance was successful in 94% of pseudocysts, even though 24% of patients had gastric varices and 48% of pseudocysts did not have a visible endoscopic bulge. Other groups have corroborated the ability to successfully perform pseudocyst drainage in the setting of portal hypertension and intervening gastric varices.[66]

Kahaleh and colleagues[61] compared non–EUS-guided transmural drainage versus EUS-guided transmural drainage in a prospective study of 99 patients. Fifty-three patients with bulging lesions without obvious portal hypertension underwent non–EUS-guided transmural drainage, and the remaining 46 patients underwent EUS-guided transmural drainage. There were no differences between the two groups in short-term success (94% vs 93%), long-term success (91% vs 84%), and complication rates (18% vs 19%).

The ideal duration of stent placement remains unclear. A study by Cahen and colleagues[62] of 92 patients identified a stent duration of greater than 6 weeks as an independent predictor of clinical success on multivariate analysis. The argument for longer stent duration is based on the assumption that time allows the formation and continued maturation of the cystenterostomy, permitting ongoing drainage and digestion of cyst contents even after stent removal. In contrast, Dhir and colleagues[43] showed that, with fully covered SEMS, stent removal after 3 weeks seemed to be safe and effective.

Fluid collections containing necrosis are associated with lower rates of clinical success and higher complication rates, likely reflecting a more acutely ill patient population and inadequate drainage with cystogastrostomy creation alone.[37,60] The presence of necrosis is also associated with a pseudocyst recurrence rate as high as 29%, compared with 9% and 12% in simple pseudocysts arising from acute and chronic pancreatitis respectively.[27] Nonetheless, several groups have described various endoscopic techniques for draining walled-off pancreatic necrosis with success rates exceeding 90%.[53,54] Therefore, in selected patients, despite the presence of necrosis, endoscopic drainage and necrosectomy can be performed successfully and should be considered as first-line treatment.

Comparison of Endoscopic, Percutaneous, and Surgical Drainage of Pancreatic Pseudocysts

Several investigations have directly compared endoscopic versus percutaneous and surgical drainage of pancreatic pseudocysts, showing lower morbidity associated with endoscopic approaches.[19,60,67]

Melman and colleagues[19] retrospectively compared the outcomes of 83 patients who underwent cystogastrostomy, of whom 22 patients underwent open cystogastrostomy, 16 underwent laparoscopic cystogastrostomy, and 45 underwent endoscopic cystogastrostomy. Significant complications occurred in 22.7% of the open surgery group, 31.5% of the laparoscopic group, and 15.6% of the endoscopic group.

The primary and overall success rates of cyst resolution were 51.1% and 84.6% for endoscopic cystogastrostomy, 87.5% and 93.8% for laparoscopic cystogastrostomy, and 81.2% and 90.9% for open cystogastrostomy. The investigators concluded that laparoscopic and open pancreatic cystogastrostomy both have a higher primary success rate than endoscopic drainage, but repeat endoscopic cystogastrostomy provides comparable overall success for selected patients.

Varadarajulu and colleagues[21,22] compared endoscopic versus surgical management in multiple investigations. An initial study compared 10 patients who underwent surgical cystogastrostomy matched against 20 patients who underwent EUS-guided cystogastrostomy,[22] whereas a subsequent study randomized 40 patients to either surgical or EUS-guided cystogastrostomy.[21] Patients with necrosis or abscesses were excluded from both investigations. In both studies, no significant differences in treatment success rates, procedural complications, or reinterventions between the two modalities were shown. However, both studies reported a significantly shorter mean length of postprocedure hospital stay with EUS-guided cystogastrostomy compared with surgical cystogastrostomy, with estimated cost savings of $5738 to $8040 per patient in the EUS-guided cystogastrostomy group. These data suggest that endoscopic cystogastrostomy achieves comparable clinical success and results in significant cost savings compared with the surgical approach, and thus is the preferred modality for pseudocyst drainage.

Percutaneous drainage has been compared with surgical drainage and shown to have an overall poor success rate with high complication rate and mortality.[68–70] Recently, in a retrospective cohort study, Akshintala and colleagues[25] compared endoscopic and percutaneous drainage in patients with symptomatic pancreatic pseudocysts. As with previous comparative studies, patients with walled-off pancreatic necrosis were excluded. A total of 81 patients were evaluated, of whom 41 underwent endoscopic drainage and 40 underwent percutaneous drainage. There were no differences in technical success, clinical success, and adverse event rates between the two groups. However, compared with those who underwent endoscopic drainage, patients who underwent percutaneous drainage had significantly higher rates of reintervention (42.5% vs 9.8%), longer length of hospital stay (14.8 vs 6.5 days), and increased number of follow-up abdominal imaging studies. Nevertheless, there remains a role for the percutaneous approach, such as in those patients who are at high risk for operative or endoscopic procedures, or patients whose pancreatic fluid collections are not amenable to endoscopic therapy.

Complications of Endoscopic Pseudocyst Drainage

Major complications of endoscopic pseudocyst drainage include lack of resolution (6%–14%), immediate or delayed bleeding (0%–9%), immediate or delayed infection (0%–8%), and retroperitoneal perforation (0%–5%).[26,29,60–63,71]

Bleeding during transmural drainage may arise from puncture of a pseudoaneurysm, gastric varices, or other vessels within the gastric or duodenal wall. Hemorrhage may be life threatening, especially in situations of inadvertent pseudoaneurysm puncture. EUS guidance during cyst entry is useful in visualizing surrounding vascular structures and therefore mitigating the risk of inadvertent vascular puncture. If EUS-guided cyst entry is not performed, preprocedural high-resolution contrast CT imaging is necessary to rule out the presence of a pseudoaneurysm. If CT findings are equivocal, Doppler ultrasonography or angiography may be used. With all non–EUS-guided cyst entry techniques, bleeding can be minimized by maintaining a steady needle position during puncture and avoiding any stroking motions of the needle knife.

Procedure-related infections may result from contamination of an incompletely drained pseudocyst caused by premature stent occlusion or uneven pseudocyst collapse. Periprocedural antimicrobial prophylaxis should be provided with a fluoro-quinolone or similar broad-spectrum antibiotic in order to reduce the incidence of pseudocyst infection.[72] Antibiotics are typically given for 3 to 5 days following pseu-docyst drainage. In addition, pancreatic necrosis significantly increases the risks for infection and failure of endoscopic drainage.[37,54,73] Serial, short-interval endoscopic necrosectomy sessions combined with intravenous antibiotics may be necessary to successfully treat infectious complications that arise from retained necrotic debris.[1]

Retroperitoneal perforation may occur when the pseudocyst wall is immature or when the distance between the pseudocyst and gut wall is greater than 1 cm.[1] Perfo-ration is a serious complication, which may result in the leakage of pseudocyst con-tents into the peritoneum and resultant peritonitis. Thus the use of guidance via EUS-guided puncture is increasingly recommended to avoid this complication.

Transpapillary stenting carries the additional risk of post-ERCP pancreatitis.[26,27] The use of indomethacin suppositories (100 mg) is recommended for all patients at high risk for this complication.[74]

SUMMARY AND APPROACH TO PANCREATIC PSEUDOCYSTS

Endoscopic drainage should be considered first-line therapy for management of pancreatic pseudocysts. Multiple endoscopic techniques have been described for pseudocyst drainage as well as irrigation and debridement of walled-off necro-sis.[21–23,59] Careful patient selection remains paramount, and exclusion of immature collections and cystic neoplasms is mandatory.

Percutaneous drainage is preferred for fluid collections that are not adjacent to the gastrointestinal lumen or do not communicate with the pancreatic duct, are immature and infected, or in patients who are poor surgical candidates.[1] Moreover, several hybrid techniques have now been described for walled-off pancreatic necrosis using a combi-nation of endoscopic and percutaneous drainage, which may mitigate the risk of cuta-neous fistula formation.[20,55–58] Surgical drainage should be reserved for situations in which regional expertise in endoscopy is not available, or when endoscopic and/or percu-taneous drainage methods fail, particularly in cases with significant pancreatic necrosis.[1]

Numerous studies have shown an excellent technical and clinical success rate for endoscopic pseudocyst drainage, regardless of route (transpapillary or transmural drainage), or EUS guidance.[6,21–23,26,27,37,44,60–65] Notably, placement of fully covered SEMS or LAMS may be associated with higher clinical success than the current stan-dard of multiple double-pigtail plastic stent placement, and merits further investiga-tion.[7,40,47] Furthermore, excellent clinical success rates have also been described in patients undergoing endoscopic drainage and debridement for walled-off necrosis, although dedicated devices remain lacking.[7,59] Regardless of the chosen drainage technique, in order to maximize clinical success, patients should be carefully selected and procedural techniques individually tailored in the context of a multidisciplinary approach.

REFERENCES

1. Samuelson AL, Shah RJ. Endoscopic management of pancreatic pseudocysts. Gastroenterol Clin North Am 2012;41:47–62.
2. Banks PA, Bollen TL, Dervenis C, et al. Classification of acute pancreatitis–2012: revision of the Atlanta classification and definitions by international consensus. Gut 2013;62:102–11.

3. Sahel J, Bastid C, Pellat B, et al. Endoscopic cystoduodenostomy of cysts of chronic calcifying pancreatitis: a report of 20 cases. Pancreas 1987;2:447–53.
4. Cremer M, Deviere J, Engelholm L. Endoscopic management of cysts and pseudocysts in chronic pancreatitis: long-term follow-up after 7 years of experience. Gastrointest Endosc 1989;35:1–9.
5. Giovannini M, Bernardini D, Seitz JF. Cystogastrotomy entirely performed under endosonography guidance for pancreatic pseudocyst: results in six patients. Gastrointest Endosc 1998;48:200–3.
6. Binmoeller KF, Weilert F, Shah JN, et al. Endosonography-guided transmural drainage of pancreatic pseudocysts using an exchange-free access device: initial clinical experience. Surg Endosc 2013;27:1835–9.
7. Shah RJ, Shah JN, Waxman I, et al. Safety and efficacy of endoscopic ultrasound-guided drainage of pancreatic fluid collections with lumen-apposing covered self-expanding metal stents. Clin Gastroenterol Hepatol 2015;13:747–52.
8. Brugge WR, Lauwers GY, Sahani D, et al. Cystic neoplasms of the pancreas. N Engl J Med 2004;351:1218–26.
9. Bradley EL, Clements JL Jr, Gonzalez AC. The natural history of pancreatic pseudocysts: a unified concept of management. Am J Surg 1979;137:135–41.
10. Vitas GJ, Sarr MG. Selected management of pancreatic pseudocysts: operative versus expectant management. Surgery 1992;111:123–30.
11. Yeo CJ, Bastidas JA, Lynch-Nyhan A, et al. The natural history of pancreatic pseudocysts documented by computed tomography. Surg Gynecol Obstet 1990;170:411–7.
12. Cheruvu CV, Clarke MG, Prentice M, et al. Conservative treatment as an option in the management of pancreatic pseudocyst. Ann R Coll Surg Engl 2003;85:313–6.
13. O'Malley VP, Cannon JP, Postier RG. Pancreatic pseudocysts: cause, therapy, and results. Am J Surg 1985;150:680–2.
14. Beebe DS, Bubrick MP, Onstad GR, et al. Management of pancreatic pseudocysts. Surg Gynecol Obstet 1984;159:562–4.
15. Gouyon B, Levy P, Ruszniewski P, et al. Predictive factors in the outcome of pseudocysts complicating alcoholic chronic pancreatitis. Gut 1997;41:821–5.
16. Nguyen BL, Thompson JS, Edney JA, et al. Influence of the etiology of pancreatitis on the natural history of pancreatic pseudocysts. Am J Surg 1991;162:527–30 [discussion: 531].
17. Bergman S, Melvin WS. Operative and nonoperative management of pancreatic pseudocysts. Surg Clin North Am 2007;87:1447–60, ix.
18. Park AE, Heniford BT. Therapeutic laparoscopy of the pancreas. Ann Surg 2002;236:149–58.
19. Melman L, Azar R, Beddow K, et al. Primary and overall success rates for clinical outcomes after laparoscopic, endoscopic, and open pancreatic cystogastrostomy for pancreatic pseudocysts. Surg Endosc 2009;23:267–71.
20. Baron TH, Kozarek RA. Endotherapy for organized pancreatic necrosis: perspectives after 20 years. Clin Gastroenterol Hepatol 2012;10:1202–7.
21. Varadarajulu S, Bang JY, Sutton BS, et al. Equal efficacy of endoscopic and surgical cystogastrostomy for pancreatic pseudocyst drainage in a randomized trial. Gastroenterology 2013;145:583–90.e1.
22. Varadarajulu S, Lopes TL, Wilcox CM, et al. EUS versus surgical cystogastrostomy for management of pancreatic pseudocysts. Gastrointest Endosc 2008;68:649–55.
23. Johnson MD, Walsh RM, Henderson JM, et al. Surgical versus nonsurgical management of pancreatic pseudocysts. J Clin Gastroenterol 2009;43:586–90.

24. Lawrence C, Howell DA, Stefan AM, et al. Disconnected pancreatic tail syndrome: potential for endoscopic therapy and results of long-term follow-up. Gastrointest Endosc 2008;67:673–9.
25. Akshintala VS, Saxena P, Zaheer A, et al. A comparative evaluation of outcomes of endoscopic versus percutaneous drainage for symptomatic pancreatic pseudocysts. Gastrointest Endosc 2014;79:921–8 [quiz: 983.e2, 983.e5].
26. Binmoeller KF, Seifert H, Walter A, et al. Transpapillary and transmural drainage of pancreatic pseudocysts. Gastrointest Endosc 1995;42:219–24.
27. Catalano MF, Geenen JE, Schmalz MJ, et al. Treatment of pancreatic pseudocysts with ductal communication by transpapillary pancreatic duct endoprosthesis. Gastrointest Endosc 1995;42:214–8.
28. Howell DA, Holbrook RF, Bosco JJ, et al. Endoscopic needle localization of pancreatic pseudocysts before transmural drainage. Gastrointest Endosc 1993;39:693–8.
29. Monkemuller KE, Baron TH, Morgan DE. Transmural drainage of pancreatic fluid collections without electrocautery using the Seldinger technique. Gastrointest Endosc 1998;48:195–200.
30. Varadarajulu S, Wilcox CM, Tamhane A, et al. Role of EUS in drainage of peripancreatic fluid collections not amenable for endoscopic transmural drainage. Gastrointest Endosc 2007;66:1107–19.
31. Fockens P, Johnson TG, van Dullemen HM, et al. Endosonographic imaging of pancreatic pseudocysts before endoscopic transmural drainage. Gastrointest Endosc 1997;46:412–6.
32. Antillon MR, Shah RJ, Stiegmann G, et al. Single-step EUS-guided transmural drainage of simple and complicated pancreatic pseudocysts. Gastrointest Endosc 2006;63:797–803.
33. Seewald S, Thonke F, Ang TL, et al. One-step, simultaneous double-wire technique facilitates pancreatic pseudocyst and abscess drainage (with videos). Gastrointest Endosc 2006;64:805–8.
34. Reddy DN, Gupta R, Lakhtakia S, et al. Use of a novel transluminal balloon accessotome in transmural drainage of pancreatic pseudocyst (with video). Gastrointest Endosc 2008;68:362–5.
35. Pfaffenbach B, Langer M, Stabenow-Lohbauer U, et al. Endosonography controlled transgastric drainage of pancreatic pseudocysts. Dtsch Med Wochenschr 1998;123:1439–42 [in German].
36. Belle S, Collet P, Post S, et al. Temporary cystogastrostomy with self-expanding metallic stents for pancreatic necrosis. Endoscopy 2010;42:493–5.
37. Baron TH, Harewood GC, Morgan DE, et al. Outcome differences after endoscopic drainage of pancreatic necrosis, acute pancreatic pseudocysts, and chronic pancreatic pseudocysts. Gastrointest Endosc 2002;56:7–17.
38. Talreja JP, Shami VM, Ku J, et al. Transenteric drainage of pancreatic-fluid collections with fully covered self-expanding metallic stents (with video). Gastrointest Endosc 2008;68:1199–203.
39. Penn DE, Draganov PV, Wagh MS, et al. Prospective evaluation of the use of fully covered self-expanding metal stents for EUS-guided transmural drainage of pancreatic pseudocysts. Gastrointest Endosc 2012;76:679–84.
40. Sharaiha RZ, DeFilippis EM, Kedia P, et al. Metal versus plastic for pancreatic pseudocyst drainage: clinical outcomes and success. Gastrointest Endosc 2015;82:822–7.
41. Yamamoto N, Isayama H, Kawakami H, et al. Preliminary report on a new, fully covered, metal stent designed for the treatment of pancreatic fluid collections. Gastrointest Endosc 2013;77:809–14.

42. Mukai S, Itoi T, Sofuni A, et al. Clinical evaluation of endoscopic ultrasonography-guided drainage using a novel flared-type biflanged metal stent for pancreatic fluid collection. Endosc Ultrasound 2015;4:120–5.

43. Dhir V, Teoh AY, Bapat M, et al. EUS-guided pseudocyst drainage: prospective evaluation of early removal of fully covered self-expandable metal stents with pancreatic ductal stenting in selected patients. Gastrointest Endosc 2015; 82(4):650–7.

44. Binmoeller KF, Shah J. A novel lumen-apposing stent for transluminal drainage of nonadherent extraintestinal fluid collections. Endoscopy 2011; 43:337–42.

45. Itoi T, Binmoeller KF, Shah J, et al. Clinical evaluation of a novel lumen-apposing metal stent for endosonography-guided pancreatic pseudocyst and gallbladder drainage (with videos). Gastrointest Endosc 2012;75:870–6.

46. Gornals JB, De la Serna-Higuera C, Sanchez-Yague A, et al. Endosonography-guided drainage of pancreatic fluid collections with a novel lumen-apposing stent. Surg Endosc 2013;27:1428–34.

47. Walter D, Will U, Sanchez-Yague A, et al. A novel lumen-apposing metal stent for endoscopic ultrasound-guided drainage of pancreatic fluid collections: a prospective cohort study. Endoscopy 2015;47:63–7.

48. Moon JH, Choi HJ, Kim DC, et al. A newly designed fully covered metal stent for lumen apposition in EUS-guided drainage and access: a feasibility study (with videos). Gastrointest Endosc 2014;79:990–5.

49. Varadarajulu S, Bang JY, Phadnis MA, et al. Endoscopic transmural drainage of peripancreatic fluid collections: outcomes and predictors of treatment success in 211 consecutive patients. J Gastrointest Surg 2011;15:2080–8.

50. Seifert H, Wehrmann T, Schmitt T, et al. Retroperitoneal endoscopic debridement for infected peripancreatic necrosis. Lancet 2000;356:653–5.

51. Seewald S, Groth S, Omar S, et al. Aggressive endoscopic therapy for pancreatic necrosis and pancreatic abscess: a new safe and effective treatment algorithm (videos). Gastrointest Endosc 2005;62:92–100.

52. Kozarek RA. Endoscopic management of pancreatic necrosis: not for the uncommitted. Gastrointest Endosc 2005;62:101–4.

53. Gardner TB, Coelho-Prabhu N, Gordon SR, et al. Direct endoscopic necrosectomy for the treatment of walled-off pancreatic necrosis: results from a multicenter U.S. series. Gastrointest Endosc 2011;73:718–26.

54. Voermans RP, Veldkamp MC, Rauws EA, et al. Endoscopic transmural debridement of symptomatic organized pancreatic necrosis (with videos). Gastrointest Endosc 2007;66:909–16.

55. Navarrete C, Castillo C, Caracci M, et al. Wide percutaneous access to pancreatic necrosis with self-expandable stent: new application (with video). Gastrointest Endosc 2011;73:609–10.

56. Gluck M, Ross A, Irani S, et al. Endoscopic and percutaneous drainage of symptomatic walled-off pancreatic necrosis reduces hospital stay and radiographic resources. Clin Gastroenterol Hepatol 2010;8:1083–8.

57. Gluck M, Ross A, Irani S, et al. Dual modality drainage for symptomatic walled-off pancreatic necrosis reduces length of hospitalization, radiological procedures, and number of endoscopies compared to standard percutaneous drainage. J Gastrointest Surg 2012;16:248–56 [discussion: 256–7].

58. Ross AS, Irani S, Gan SI, et al. Dual-modality drainage of infected and symptomatic walled-off pancreatic necrosis: long-term clinical outcomes. Gastrointest Endosc 2014;79:929–35.

59. Varadarajulu S, Phadnis MA, Christein JD, et al. Multiple transluminal gateway technique for EUS-guided drainage of symptomatic walled-off pancreatic necrosis. Gastrointest Endosc 2011;74:74–80.
60. Hookey LC, Debroux S, Delhaye M, et al. Endoscopic drainage of pancreatic-fluid collections in 116 patients: a comparison of etiologies, drainage techniques, and outcomes. Gastrointest Endosc 2006;63:635–43.
61. Kahaleh M, Shami VM, Conaway MR, et al. Endoscopic ultrasound drainage of pancreatic pseudocyst: a prospective comparison with conventional endoscopic drainage. Endoscopy 2006;38:355–9.
62. Cahen D, Rauws E, Fockens P, et al. Endoscopic drainage of pancreatic pseudocysts: long-term outcome and procedural factors associated with safe and successful treatment. Endoscopy 2005;37:977–83.
63. Weckman L, Kylanpaa ML, Puolakkainen P, et al. Endoscopic treatment of pancreatic pseudocysts. Surg Endosc 2006;20:603–7.
64. Giovannini M, Pesenti C, Rolland AL, et al. Endoscopic ultrasound-guided drainage of pancreatic pseudocysts or pancreatic abscesses using a therapeutic echo endoscope. Endoscopy 2001;33:473–7.
65. Barthet M, Sahel J, Bodiou-Bertei C, et al. Endoscopic transpapillary drainage of pancreatic pseudocysts. Gastrointest Endosc 1995;42:208–13.
66. Sriram PV, Kaffes AJ, Rao GV, et al. Endoscopic ultrasound-guided drainage of pancreatic pseudocysts complicated by portal hypertension or by intervening vessels. Endoscopy 2005;37:231–5.
67. Rosso E, Alexakis N, Ghaneh P, et al. Pancreatic pseudocyst in chronic pancreatitis: endoscopic and surgical treatment. Dig Surg 2003;20:397–406.
68. Heider R, Meyer AA, Galanko JA, et al. Percutaneous drainage of pancreatic pseudocysts is associated with a higher failure rate than surgical treatment in unselected patients. Ann Surg 1999;229:781–7 [discussion: 787–9].
69. Adams DB, Anderson MC. Percutaneous catheter drainage compared with internal drainage in the management of pancreatic pseudocyst. Ann Surg 1992;215:571–6 [discussion: 576–8].
70. Morton JM, Brown A, Galanko JA, et al. A national comparison of surgical versus percutaneous drainage of pancreatic pseudocysts: 1997-2001. J Gastrointest Surg 2005;9:15–20 [discussion: 20–1].
71. Kruger M, Schneider AS, Manns MP, et al. Endoscopic management of pancreatic pseudocysts or abscesses after an EUS-guided 1-step procedure for initial access. Gastrointest Endosc 2006;63:409–16.
72. Khashab MA, Chithadi KV, Jiang B. Antibiotic prophylaxis for GI endoscopy. Gastrointest Endosc 2015;81:81–9.
73. Hariri M, Slivka A, Carr-Locke DL, et al. Pseudocyst drainage predisposes to infection when pancreatic necrosis is unrecognized. Am J Gastroenterol 1994;89:1781–4.
74. Elmunzer BJ, Scheiman JM, Lehman GA, et al. A randomized trial of rectal indomethacin to prevent post-ERCP pancreatitis. N Engl J Med 2012;366:1414–22.

Autoimmune Pancreatitis
An Update on Diagnosis and Management

Kamraan Madhani, MD[a], James J. Farrell, MD[b],*

KEYWORDS

- Autoimmune pancreatitis • Lymphoplasmacytic sclerosing pancreatitis
- Idiopathic duct-centric pancreatitis • IgG4
- International Consensus Diagnostic Criteria • Corticosteroids

KEY POINTS

- Autoimmune pancreatitis (AIP) can affect the pancreas primarily; however, it can also present as part of a systemic disease related to immunoglobulin G4.
- AIP is primarily a histologic diagnosis, but AIP is currently diagnosed using clinical characteristics.
- The mainstay of therapy for AIP is corticosteroids. Other therapies that have been explored include immunomodulator drugs.
- Relapse rates following corticosteroid therapy are high.

INTRODUCTION

Cases of autoimmune pancreatitis (AIP) were described as early as the 1960s by Sarles and colleagues.[1] However, the term autoimmune pancreatitis was first introduced by Yoshida and colleagues[2] in 1995 after these investigators studied a Japanese cohort with causes suggestive of autoimmune origin. Although AIP is recognized as a distinct disease process, the incidence remains unknown. A 2009 survey in Japan estimated that the incidence of AIP in the Ishikawa district (population 1.16 million) was approximately 1 per 100,000.[3] The rate of undiagnosed AIP in large cohorts of patients undergoing pancreatic surgical resection of presumed pancreatic cancer is approximately 2%.[4,5]

AIP was initially recognized as a disease associated with characteristic clinical, radiologic, and serologic features affecting primarily the pancreas, with the ability to

Disclosure: The authors have nothing to disclose.
[a] Yale-Waterbury Internal Medicine Residency Program, Yale University School of Medicine, New Haven, CT 06510, USA; [b] Yale Center for Pancreatic Disease, Section of Digestive Disease, Yale University, LMP 1080, 15 York Street, New Haven, CT 06510, USA
* Corresponding author.
E-mail address: james.j.farrell@yale.edu

Gastroenterol Clin N Am 45 (2016) 29–43
http://dx.doi.org/10.1016/j.gtc.2015.10.005
0889-8553/16/$ – see front matter © 2016 Elsevier Inc. All rights reserved.

involve other organs. However, more recently AIP has been associated with other immune-mediated diseases, including immunoglobulin (Ig) G4–associated cholangitis (IAC), salivary gland disorders, mediastinal fibrosis, retroperitoneal fibrosis, tubulointerstitial disease and inflammatory bowel disease, and increased levels of IgG4, both in tissue plasma cells and in the serum,[6] thus terming this collection of disease processes IgG4-related systemic disease.

With improved understanding of AIP and its distinct clinical profiles and variable association with a systemic IgG4 disease process, AIP has been classified into type 1 and type 2 AIP. In type 1 AIP, the pancreas is affected as part of a systemic IgG4-positive disease, also known as lymphoplasmacytic sclerosing pancreatitis (LPSP). Type 2 AIP is characterized by histologically confirmed idiopathic duct-centric pancreatitis, often with granulocytic epithelial lesions (GELs) with or without granulocytic acinar inflammation along with absent (0–10 cells per high-power field [HPF]) IgG4-positive cells, and without systemic involvement. Classic clinical characteristics include obstructive jaundice, abdominal pain, and acute pancreatitis, which make exclusion of pancreatic cancer necessary before the diagnosis of AIP. However, unlike pancreatic malignancies, AIP may respond to therapy with corticosteroids.

Although AIP is primarily a pathologic diagnosis, attempts have been made to clinically diagnose AIP using various clinical criteria. In 2011 an international symposium on AIP yielded the International Consensus Diagnostic Criteria (ICDC),[7] which can be used to classify AIP as type 1, type 2, or AIP–Not Otherwise Specified. This article discusses clinical, pathologic, and serologic features of AIP with mention of the various diagnostic guidelines that have been used to diagnose AIP, with a special focus on ICDC. Management options are also discussed.

Clinical Characteristics

Patients with type I AIP typically present at an older age (on average 16 years older) than patients presenting with type 2 AIP.[8] Patients with either type of AIP commonly present with obstructive jaundice, abdominal pain, and/or biochemical evidence of pancreatitis. The study of a large cohort of 731 patients found that obstructive jaundice was the presenting symptom in 75% of patients with type 1 AIP compared with abdominal pain being the most common presentation in 68% of patients with type 2 AIP.[8] The obstructive jaundice may be related to pancreatic swelling and compression of the biliary tree, or be caused by proximal extrahepatic and intrahepatic duct stricture, which can be part of an associated IAC.[9] The abdominal pain is typically mild and may or may not be associated with documented attacks of acute pancreatitis. AIP is not a common cause for idiopathic recurrent pancreatitis. Increases in IgG4 levels are typically seen more often with type 1 AIP, with the degree of increase in IgG4 level necessary to satisfy level 1 evidence for the diagnosis of type 1 AIP greater than twice the upper limit of normal. A level less than twice the upper limit of normal is consistent with level 2 evidence per ICDC guidelines.[7] Imaging findings range from either diffuse or focal pancreatic involvement, often with evidence of other organ involvement (OOI), including hilar lymphadenopathy, extrapancreatic biliary duct involvement, or renal masses. Type 1 AIP is more likely to have biliary tract disease and a higher rate of relapse compared with type 2 AIP.[10]

Diagnostic Guidelines

Because therapy and prognosis differ greatly between the two diseases, exclusion of pancreatic adenocarcinoma must be confirmed before pursuing AIP as a diagnosis. It is also important to diagnose AIP because treatment may avert the long-term consequences of the disease, in addition to avoiding unnecessary surgery.

Numerous guidelines have evolved to reasonably differentiate AIP from pancreatic cancer preoperatively using methods that are noninvasive, such as imaging, serology, and trial with steroid therapy. These clinical guidelines include the Japanese Pancreas Society (JPS; JPS-2006,[11] JPS-2011[12]), Korean Criteria,[13] Asian Criteria,[14] HISORt (histology, imaging, serology, OOI, response to corticosteroids),[15] and most recently the ICDC.[7]

The Japanese Pancreas Society guidelines

The JPS originally published diagnostic guidelines in 2002, which have since been revised in 2006[11] and 2011.[12] With JPS-2006,[11] the diagnosis of AIP can be made by 2 possible methods, both requiring imaging. With the addition of serology (showing increased levels of gamma globulins or immunoglobulins) or histology (showing LPSP), diagnosis can be confirmed.

In 2011 these guidelines were revised to yield JPS-2011[12] to provide more avenues for reaching a diagnosis. The main difference between JPS-2011[12] and any other diagnostic guidelines is the requirement for diagnostic endoscopic retrograde cholangiopancreatography (ERCP; pancreatogram) in any patient with atypical parenchymal imaging.[12] Without ERCP, the diagnosis of definitive, probable, or possible AIP is impossible with these guidelines. The reason for mandatory ERCP in such cases is to avoid misdiagnosis of pancreatic cancer.[12] For those patients who have typical findings of AIP on parenchymal imaging the diagnosis can be made with the addition of serology, OOI, or histology.

The HISORt guidelines

The HISORt[15] criteria, originating from the Mayo Clinic in 2006, are based on a mnemonic that can be used to recall diagnostic features of AIP. These features include:

1. Histology (H)
2. Imaging (P-Parenchymal; D-Ductal)
3. Serology (S)
4. OOI
5. Response to corticosteroids (Rt)

Considering the available features, patients can meet the diagnosis with evidence of diagnostic histology, typical imaging and serology, or response to corticosteroids.

The Korean and Asian guidelines

The Asian[14] guidelines, formulated in 2008, represent a collaboration between the Japanese[11] and Korean[13] guidelines. Unlike JPS-2006,[11] the Korean[13] guidelines adopted OOI and response to corticosteroid therapy in their guidelines. With the Korean[13] guidelines, OOI or response to steroid therapy can be paired with parenchymal or ductal imaging to diagnose AIP. However, the resulting Asian[14] guidelines concluded that imaging, serology, and histology could be considered as acceptable evidence for diagnosis, and corticosteroid response could be used as an optional collateral piece of data. Hence the definitive diagnosis of AIP is possible with the combination of imaging with either serology or histology only, using these guidelines.

The International Consensus Diagnostic Criteria guidelines

In 2011, an international panel of experts met during the 14th Congress of the International Association of Pancreatology and developed the ICDC (**Tables 1 and 2**).[7] The significance of these guidelines is they allowed for flexibility in the diagnosis of both subtypes of AIP and can be used in clinical and research practice. Unlike older criteria, they do not require typical pancreatic imaging in order to make the diagnosis, instead

Table 1
Level 1 and level 2 criteria for type 1 AIP for the ICDC

Diagnosis	Primary Basis for Diagnosis	Imaging Evidence	Collateral Evidence
Definitive type 1 AIP	Histology	Typical/indeterminate	Histologically confirmed LPSP (level 1 H)
	Imaging	Typical	Any non-D level 1/level 2
		Indeterminate	Two or more from level 1 (+ level 2 D[a])
	Response to steroid	Indeterminate	Level 1 S/OOI + Rt or level 1 D + level 2 S/OOI/H + Rt
Probable type 1 AIP	—	Indeterminate	Level 2 S/OOI/H + Rt

[a] Level 2 D is counted as level 1 in this setting.
From Shimosegawa T, Chari ST, Frulloni L, et al. International Consensus Diagnostic Criteria for autoimmune pancreatitis: guidelines of the International Association of Pancreatology. Pancreas 2011;40(3):353; with permission.

providing multiple avenues that can be taken, depending on available data, in order to make definite or probable diagnosis of AIP.

Typically, the first step is to evaluate parenchymal imaging and categorize it as either typical (level 1) or atypical (level 2). Typical characteristics on parenchymal imaging include diffuse enlargement with delayed enhancement, sometimes associated with a rimlike enhancement. Segmental enlargement or delayed enhancement meets atypical or level 2 criteria.[7] Depending on which level of evidence is present, the requirements for supporting evidence vary. For example, patients who have typical/level 1 parenchymal imaging on computed tomography (CT) or MRI would then undergo evaluation for OOI and serum measurement of IgG4 level. If either of these criteria meets level 1 or level 2 evidence, then this would be highly suggestive of type 1 AIP. Patients such as this would then be considered for treatment with corticosteroids. In contrast, in patients who have atypical/level 2 parenchymal imaging, if neither OOI nor serology meet typical/level 1 criteria then an endoscopic pancreatogram and pancreatic biopsy are required in order to proceed with the diagnosis of type 1 AIP.[7]

The ICDC[7] use the 5 cardinal features of AIP:

1. Pancreatic imaging of either parenchyma or ducts
2. Serology
3. OOI
4. Histology of the pancreas
5. Response to corticosteroid therapy (Rt)

Details regarding each of these cardinal features as they pertain to ICDC[7] are discussed later.

Pancreatic imaging Pancreatic imaging abnormalities are found in up to 85% of patients with AIP.[16] Features suggestive of AIP on CT or MRI are diffuse parenchymal enlargement with delayed enhancement, sometimes associated with rimlike enhancement (**Fig. 1**). Indeterminate imaging of the pancreas includes segmental or focal enlargement with delayed enhancement.[7] Peripancreatic vascular involvement is rarely described, and can be confused with features of locally advanced malignancy.[16,17] Endoscopic ultrasonography (EUS) and transabdominal ultrasonography have also been used to evaluate the parenchyma of the pancreas (**Fig. 2**).[17,18]

Table 2
Diagnosis of definitive and probable type 1 AIP using ICDC

	Criterion	Level 1	Level 2
P	Parenchymal imaging	Typical: diffuse enlargement with delayed enhancement (sometimes associated with rimlike enhancement)	Indeterminate (including atypical[b]): segmental/focal enlargement with delayed enhancement
D	Ductal imaging (ERP)	Long (>one-third length of the main pancreatic duct) or multiple strictures without marked upstream dilatation	Segmental/focal narrowing without marked upstream dilatation (duct size <5 mm)
S	Serology	IgG4 level >2 × upper limit of normal	IgG4 level 1–2 × upper limit of normal

OOI	Other organ involvement	a or b
		a. Histology of extrapancreatic organs
		 Any 3 of the following:
		  1. Marked lymphoplasmacytic infiltration with fibrosis and without granulocytic infiltration
		  2. Storiform fibrosis
		  3. Obliterative phlebitis
		  4. Abundant (>l0 cells/HPF) IgG4-positive cells
		b. Typical radiologic evidence
		 At least 1 of the following:
		  1. Segmental/multiple proximal (hilar/intrahepatic) or proximal and distal bile duct stricture
		  2. Retroperitoneal fibrosis
			a or b
			a. Histology of extrapancreatic organs including endoscopic biopsies of bile duct[c]:
			 Both of the following:
			  1. Marked lymphoplasmacytic infiltration without granulocytic infiltration
			  2. Abundant (>10 cells/HPF) IgG4-positive cells
			b. Physical or radiologic evidence
			 At least 1 of the following:
			  1. Symmetrically enlarged salivary/lachrymal glands
			  2. Radiologic evidence of renal involvement described in association with AIP

H	Histology of the pancreas	LPSP (core biopsy/resection)
		 At least 3 of the following:
		  1. Periductal lymphoplasmacytic infiltrate without granulocytic infiltration
		  2. Obliterative phlebitis
		  3. Storiform fibrosis
		  4. Abundant (>l0 cells/HPF) IgG4-positive cells
			LPSP (core biopsy)
			 Any 2 of the following:
			  1. Periductal lymphoplasmacytic infiltrate without granulocytic infiltration
			  2. Obliterative phlebitis
			  3. Stoiform fibrosis
			  4. Abundant (>10 cells/HPF) IgG4-positive cells

Rt[a]	Diagnostic steroid trial Rapid (≤2 wk) radiologically demonstrable resolution or marked improvement in pancreatic/extrapancreatic manifestations		

Abbreviations: ERP, endoscopic retrograde pancreatography; Rt, response to corticosteroid therapy.

[a] Diagnostic steroid trial should be conducted carefully by pancreatologists with caveats (see text) only after negative work-up for cancer, including endoscopic ultrasonography-guided fine-needle aspiration.

[b] Atypical: AIP cases may show low-density mass, pancreatic ductal dilatation, or distal atrophy. Such atypical imaging findings in patients with obstructive jaundice and/or pancreatic mass are highly suggestive of pancreatic cancer. Such patients should be managed as having pancreatic cancer unless there is strong collateral evidence for AIP, and a thorough work-up for cancer is negative (see algorithm).

[c] Endoscopic biopsy of duodenal papilla is a useful adjunctive method because ampullae are often involved pathologically in AIP.

From Shimosegawa T, Chari ST, Frulloni L, et al. International Consensus Diagnostic Criteria for autoimmune pancreatitis: guidelines of the International Association of Pancreatology. Pancreas 2011;40(3):354; with permission.

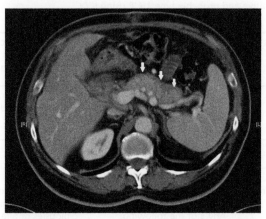

Fig. 1. Contrast-enhanced CT scan shows diffuse enlargement of the pancreas with sharp borders and minimal peripancreatic stranding (*arrows*). The hypoenhancing rim (the halo) is strongly suggestive of AIP.

A recent prospective study compared 32 patients with AIP with a control population of patients with pancreatic adenocarcinoma based on CT imaging features. Independently, 3 radiologists read the images and reported common features seen in each disease. The most common findings seen on CT in patients with AIP were common bile duct (CBD) stricture (63%), bile duct wall hyperenhancement (47%), and diffuse parenchymal enlargement (41%). In contrast, in the control population the most common CT imaging features were focal mass (78%) and pancreatic ductal dilatation (69%). In 10 patients with pathologically confirmed AIP, the misdiagnosis of pancreatic adenocarcinoma was made based on radiology primarily because of the presence of a focal mass, which was seen in 9 patients (90%).[19] A similar study compared 101 patients with AIP, pancreatic carcinoma, and control patients without AIP or pancreatic

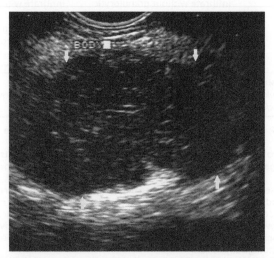

Fig. 2. EUS imaging of the pancreas in AIP shows profound hypoechoic infiltration of the pancreas body. Normal-sized pancreatic duct is shown (*arrows*).

cancer.[20] This study showed that under dual-phase CT scan, the enhancement patterns differ between patients with AIP and those with pancreatic cancer and normal pancreas samples. Features typical for AIP have also been described with the use of multiple detector CT, with the most common features suggestive of AIP being a sausage shape (64%) and low-attenuation halo (59%).[21] Thus, findings on CT that are atypical for AIP should prompt investigation for alternative diagnosis.[17]

ERCP and magnetic resonance cholangiography ductal imaging features, although limited on their own, can provide useful collateral evidence in diagnosing AIP in cases in which parenchymal imaging is noncontributory. Per the ICDC[7] guidelines, typical features on ERCP are long (>one-third the length of the main pancreatic duct) or multiple strictures of the pancreatic duct without marked upstream dilatation (**Fig. 3**). Indeterminate ERCP features are segmental/focal narrowing of the main pancreatic duct without marked upstream dilatation (duct size <5 mm). Features most agreed on in diagnosing AIP in an international multicenter study were long (one-third the length of the pancreatic duct) stricture, no upstream dilatation, multiple strictures, and side branches arising from a strictured segment.[22] Similarly, a focal stricture of the proximal or distal CBD or irregular narrowing of the intrahepatic ducts can be found. However, pancreatic ductal imaging with ERCP is limited because of the limited role for diagnostic ERCP in clinical practice.

Parenchymal and ductal imaging can serve complimentary roles in establishing a diagnosis of AIP using the ICDC guidelines. Depending on which level of evidence is met, various pathways to diagnosis can be taken. When typical imaging is detected, any nonductal imaging (serology, OOI, corticosteroid therapy) evidence can be used to confirm the diagnosis of definitive AIP and invasive testing with fine-needle aspiration (FNA) biopsy or pancreas histology is not required. However, if atypical imaging is present then the diagnosis hinges on the availability of collateral evidence (see **Table 1**). The key difference that allowed improved utility of ICDC[7] compared with older guidelines was the removal of the requirement of typical imaging findings. Without typical pancreatic imaging, the diagnosis of AIP using the JPS-2006,[11] Korean,[13] and Asian[14] guidelines is not possible.

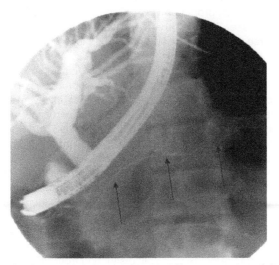

Fig. 3. ERCP shows focal stricture in distal CBD with diffuse narrowing of the pancreatic duct without upstream dilatation (*arrows*).

Serology IgG4 typically accounts for less than 5% of all the total serum IgG in normal individuals and the level is typically less than 140 mg/dL. Increases in IgG4 or serum antinuclear antibody (ANA) levels can be expected in patients with AIP.[7] Level 1 evidence is defined by at least a 2-fold increase in serum IgG4 level, and increase between 1 and 2 times the upper limit of normal satisfies level 2 evidence (see **Table 1**). This cutoff was chosen because up to 10% of individuals with pancreatic ductal cancer have values less than the 2-fold threshold.

In one study, patients with AIP had high serum concentrations of IgG4, suggesting that increased levels of these immunoglobulins were useful in evaluating patients suspected of having AIP.[6] By evaluating patients with AIP and comparing them with age-matched and sex-matched patients who were normal, the median IgG4 level in patients with AIP was 663 mg/dL compared with 51 mg/dL in normal patients. In a separate cohort,[23] 45 patients with AIP had a mean serum IgG4 level of 550 mg/dL compared with 69.5 mg/dL among 135 patients with pancreatic cancer. Furthermore, serum IgG4 levels were increased in 13 of 135 (10%) the patients with pancreatic cancer but only 1% of this group had IgG4 levels greater than 280 mg/dL, compared with 53% of the AIP subset. An IgG4 level greater than 280 mg/dL corresponds with a sensitivity and specificity of 53% and 99%, respectively. Comparatively, an IgG4 level greater than 140 mg/dl has sensitivity and specificity of 76% and 93%, respectively.

However, increases in IgG4 titers are not specific to AIP and can also be seen in pancreatic cancer.[7] Therefore, reliance on serology alone is an unwise practice and the presence of serology data should be used in tandem with other clinical and diagnostic features. However, there may be a role for IgG4 in monitoring response to medical treatment. Among 12 patients with sclerosing pancreatitis (AIP), serum IgG4 values were measured before corticosteroid therapy and after 4 weeks of therapy. Before therapy, the average IgG4 value in this group was 742 mg/dL compared with 223 mg/dL after 4 weeks, suggesting its role in monitoring treatment response.[6] Antibodies measured in patients with AIP, including anti–plasminogen-binding protein carbonic anhydrase II antigen and lactoferrin, do not have sufficient sensitivity and specificity to separate out AIP from pancreatic malignancy.[24–26]

Other organ involvement Given the myriad of extrapancreatic manifestations possible in AIP, it has been proposed that AIP is part of a systemic process caused by IgG4-related disease. The extrapancreatic sites that are commonly involved include the biliary tree, lacrimal and salivary glands, as well as the kidneys, retroperitoneum, pituitary, and prostate.[27,28] In type 1 AIP, OOI can be detected on radiology or histology. Radiologic evidence showing segmental/multiple proximal (hilar/intrahepatic) or proximal and distal bile duct stricture, retroperitoneal fibrosis, symmetrically enlarged salivary or lachrymal glands, or evidence of renal involvement can all be used to meet either level of evidence for type 1 AIP. Extrapancreatic organs showing evidence of marked lymphoplasmacytic infiltration with fibrosis and without granulocytic infiltration, with storiform fibrosis, obliterative phlebitis, or abundant (>10 cells/HPF) IgG4-positive cells can be used to show histologic OOI.[7]

Initially, AIP was thought to be associated with primary sclerosing cholangitis (PSC); however, the intrahepatic and extrahepatic biliary tract abnormalities with stricture seen in AIP are most often related to an IAC, often with associated increases of serum IgG4 levels.[29] PSC biliary strictures are typically bandlike with a beaded or pruned appearance, whereas IACs are typically segmental, long strictures with a prestenotic dilatation, and are more commonly seen in the distal CBD. AIP-related biliary strictures are more likely to respond to steroids.[30,31] This distinction from PSC has been confirmed by a pathology study of gallbladders from patients with AIP, PSC, and pancreatic carcinoma. There were dense extramural infiltrates in 41% of gallbladders of patients with AIP, compared with only 4% of patients with pancreatic carcinoma and 0% in patients with PSC. In addition, specimens from patients with AIP showed a higher IgG4/IgG ratio compared with PSC and pancreatic carcinoma counterparts.[28,29,32]

Bowel involvement is primarily associated with type 2 AIP; however, there are reports of patients with type 1 AIP concurrently diagnosed with inflammatory bowel disease. According to a multicenter international study that compared 204 patients with type 1 AIP and 64 patients with type 2 AIP, patients with type 2 AIP were more likely to have concurrent inflammatory bowel disease, specifically ulcerative colitis: 16% versus 1%, respectively.[8]

Histology The characteristic histologic feature of type 1 AIP is LPSP, whereas type 2 AIP, also known as idiopathic duct-centric pancreatitis (IDCP), is more classically associated with GELs with or without granulocytic acinar inflammation, along with absent (0–10 cells/HPF) IgG4-positive cells (**Fig. 4**). However, GELs are not specific for type 2 AIP, and may be found in 27% of type 1 AIP cases.[33]

In addition to the histologic evidence of periductal lymphoplasmacytic infiltrate without granulocytic infiltration, at least 2 additional histologic features are required in order to meet level 1 evidence for type 1 AIP. Features that may be combined to make a diagnosis include obliterative phlebitis, storiform fibrosis, and abundant (>10 cells/HPF) IgG4-positive cells. The presence of just 1 additional feature meets the criteria for level 2 evidence.[7]

Unlike type 1 AIP, type 2 AIP requires tissue to confirm the diagnosis per the ICDC guidelines. Lack of association of IDCP with increased levels of IgG4 and OOI requires tissue in order to avoid the misdiagnosis of pancreatic malignancy as AIP. However, obtaining a histologic diagnosis in the absence of surgical resection is challenging. There is too little experience with either EUS-guided or radiology-guided FNA or core biopsies of pancreas to obtain sufficient cytologic or histologic tissue to make a diagnosis (**Fig. 5**).[17,34–36] The additional immunostaining for IgG4 in extrapancreatic tissue may also support the diagnosis of AIP.[37]

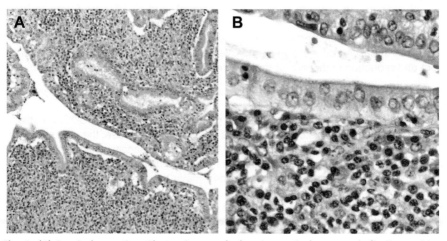

Fig. 4. (*A*) Surgical resection. Photomicrograph showing typical pancreatic findings with a heavy periductal lymphocytic and plasmacytic infiltration around the pancreatic ducts. There is a lesser degree of neutrophilic inflammation in duct lumens (hematoxylin-eosin [H&E], original magnification × 40). (*B*) Higher power photomicrograph showing periductal infiltration (H&E, original magnification × 100).

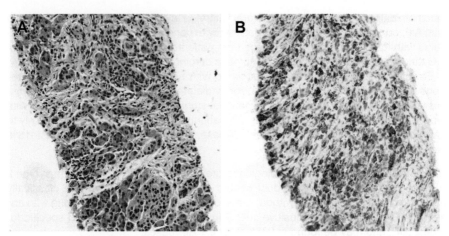

Fig. 5. (*A*) Pancreatic histologic core biopsy showing AIP using EUS FNA biopsy (H&E ×40). (*B*) Pancreatic histologic core biopsy showing IgG4 immunostaining of plasma cells in AIP using EUS FNA biopsy (H&E ×40).

Diagnostic trial of corticosteroids Only after pancreatic malignancy has been ruled out, including a negative EUS-guided FNA, should a diagnostic steroid trial be conducted.[7] For a diagnostic corticosteroid trial to be considered positive, a rapid (within 2 weeks) improvement in radiologic pancreatic/extrapancreatic manifestations should be shown. The spontaneous resolution of symptoms or radiologic features in patients with AIP in the absence of steroid treatment, which is occasionally seen, is not considered a diagnostic criteria per the ICDC guidelines. Overall, improvement in symptoms or decreased levels of cancer antigen (CA) 19-9 should not be taken as the sole piece of evidence in the diagnosis of AIP in the absence of other diagnostic features.

The role of a diagnostic 2-week steroid trial was evaluated in 22 patients with atypical parenchymal imaging for AIP not yet differentiated from pancreatic cancer.[38] Of the 22 patients, 15 patients showed improvement, and all 15 were found to have AIP. The remaining 7 who did not improve all had pancreatic cancer, supporting the concept that a 2-week steroid trial may be helpful in confirming a diagnosis of AIP, especially in cases that resulted in improvement in narrowing of the main pancreatic duct and reduction in the size of the pancreatic mass.

Evaluation of the International Consensus Diagnostic Criteria and other diagnostic criteria

The validation of these clinical diagnostic guidelines, including the ICDC, is difficult owing to the need for a histologic diagnosis to confirm the disease: the gold standard.

Two recent validation studies comparing the diagnostic sensitivity and specificity of the 5 major criteria using a cohort of patients with AIP and control groups with pancreatic cancer showed that the ICDC guidelines[7] have the greatest sensitivity (90.9%–95.1%) compared with Korean[13] (90.2%), JPS-2011[12] (86.9%), Asian[14] (83.6%), and HISORt[15] (83.6%), as well as the greatest specificity (up to 97%).[12,33] Thus, ICDC[7] is considered to be the most useful set of guidelines in the diagnosis of AIP.

Therapy

Corticosteroids

Corticosteroid therapy has been accepted as the mainstay of therapy for AIP, both in terms of improving symptoms and preventing long-term consequences. The standard dose typically involves 0.6 mg/kg to 1 mg/kg for 2 to 4 weeks with a taper of 5 mg/d every week. Markers to follow during treatment with corticosteroids include resolution of symptoms; repeat imaging with CT or MRI; and trending of CA 19-9, liver function tests, and IgG4 levels.

Early corticosteroid therapy is indicated in patients with AIP unless otherwise contraindicated.[39] In a cohort study of 42 patients with AIP, 23 patients were observed without corticosteroid therapy and 19 patients were administered corticosteroid therapy. After an average observation period of 25 months, 70% of those without corticosteroid therapy had unfavorable events, which were defined as obstructive jaundice, pancreatic pseudocyst, sclerogenic changes of extrapancreatic bile ducts, hydronephrosis, or interstitial nephritis, compared with only 32% of those who were treated with corticosteroid therapy.[39]

To establish an appropriate steroid regimen, a multicenter study in Japan retrospectively studied a cohort of 459 patients who were treated with prednisolone at 0.6 mg/kg. They recorded a remission rate of 98% among this treatment group compared with a remission rate of 74% of patients who were not treated with corticosteroids. In this same study, maintenance therapy with corticosteroids was administered in 377 patients (82%) and the relapse rate among those on maintenance therapy was 23%, compared with 34% in patients who were not continued on maintenance therapy.[40] The difference in outcomes between low-dose (10 mg/d) and high-dose (60 mg/d) corticosteroid therapy has been reported to be similar.[41]

Until recently there were few studies that evaluated the long-term response to therapy with corticosteroids. A large multinational study of more than 1000 patients, including 978 with type 1 AIP and 86 with type 2 AIP, found that 99% of patients with type 1 AIP and 92% of patients with type 2 went into remission after being treated with steroids. Indications for steroid therapy in this cohort included jaundice (63% type 1 and 25% type 2) and pancreatitis/abdominal pain (27% type 1 and 64% type 2). Some other indications for steroid therapy include abnormal imaging, salivary gland enlargement, and diagnostic steroid trial.[42] However, on discontinuation of steroids, relapses were a common occurrence in up to 31% of patients with type 1 and 9% of patients with type 2.

Although most patients initially response to steroids, a large percentage of patients relapse once steroids are discontinued. It is not clear how long steroids should be maintained. In a study that followed patients treated with corticosteroids for AIP, relapse was detected in 12 (27%) of the patients after a median delay of 6 months. Factors associated with a high relapse rate after discontinuation of steroids included high levels of IgG4 at the time of diagnosis and OOI, including IAC.[43] Other clinical, radiologic, and pathologic factors suggesting steroid responsiveness and relapse likelihood have been suggested but require further validation. Radiologic factors predictive of a favorable response include diffuse swelling with a halo (a hypoattenuating rim surrounding the pancreas) on CT, whereas factors predicting a suboptimal response include ductal stricture and a persistent focal mass swelling after resolution of diffuse changes. Pathologically it is hypothesized that an early inflammatory phase is associated with a favorable response to corticosteroid treatment, and that a suboptimal response may be associated with tissue fibrosis.[43]

Immunomodulator drugs

The presence of other autoimmune disorders in patients with AIP and IAC, such as rheumatoid arthritis or Sjögren syndrome, supports the underlying role of B-cell activity and prompted the consideration for the use of immunomodulator therapy in patients with AIP.[44] Immunomodulator agents (eg, azathioprine, 6-mercaptopurine, rituximab, cyclosporine, and cyclophosphamide) have been used in patients with AIP who relapse following steroid withdrawal, fail steroid trial, or do not tolerate steroids. Rituximab's mechanism of action further supports that B lymphocytes and CD20 antigen play a central role in the pathogenesis of IAC.

Patients with OOI, specifically with involvement of the biliary tree (who are known to be more prone to relapses, for unclear reasons), may benefit from treatment with immunomodulation should steroid therapy be ineffective or not tolerated. Patients with IAC who cannot be weaned from steroid therapy may benefit from either combined therapy with steroids and azathioprine or with azathioprine alone.[45]

Although there are no randomized studies on the subject, in pooled data from 3 treatment studies of patients with AIP or IgG4-associated cholangitis (IAC) the overall relapse rate in patients treated with corticosteroids ranged from 27%[16] to 53%. Patients who relapsed after steroid withdrawal or failed steroid wean were retreated either with steroids or with a combination of steroids with either azathioprine or cyclophosphamide.[9,45] Immunomodulator therapies seem to be effective in patients who relapse following steroid withdrawal or who cannot tolerate being weaned off steroids; however, no large-scale studies are available and further prospective evaluation is required in this area.

In a study comparing subsequent relapse-free survival in patients who initially relapsed following steroid withdrawal and were then treated with another course of steroids alone or steroids in combination with an immunomodulator, the time to the second relapse was similar for both groups.[46] In the same study, 12 patients who could not tolerate steroids or immunomodulatory therapy were given rituximab, with 10 (83%) achieving full remission without relapse while on maintenance therapy. The use of rituximab has been reported with some success in achieving remission, but the duration of therapy, the dose, the long-term effects, and the benefits of maintenance therapy have yet to be studied, and require further evaluation.[47]

In a separate cohort of 210 patients with type 1 AIP who relapsed following steroid discontinuation or taper, treatment with another course of steroids was successful in achieving remission in 201 of 210 (95%). Azathioprine was given in conjunction with steroids in 68 patients, and achieved remission in 56 (82%). A similar remission rate of 86% was seen in a smaller subset of patients treated with mycophenolate mofetil, cyclosporine, methotrexate, 6-mercaptopurine, and cyclophosphamide.[42]

SUMMARY

Several international groups have evaluated AIP in an effort to produce diagnostic guidelines that can be applied universally by specialists and nonspecialists alike. The advent of the ICDC guidelines in 2011 represents the most current comprehensive guidelines for use in the diagnosis of AIP. The ICDC, similar to the preceding guidelines, cited the 5 cardinal features of AIP and drew on evidence from each of those features in the diagnosis of AIP. Other than histologic confirmation, the use of evidence from a single cardinal feature should not be used in isolation and instead should be paired with other evidence as outlined by ICDC in the diagnosis of AIP. Although steroids remain the mainstay of treatment of patients diagnosed with AIP, further refinements about the dose, duration, and likelihood of relapse and alternative therapies have not been adequately studied.

REFERENCES

1. Sarles H, Sarles JC, Camatte R, et al. Observations on 205 confirmed cases of acute pancreatitis, recurring pancreatitis, and chronic pancreatitis. Gut 1965; 6(6):545–59.

2. Yoshida K, Toki F, Takeuchi T, et al. Chronic pancreatitis caused by an autoimmune abnormality. Proposal of the concept of autoimmune pancreatitis. Dig Dis Sci 1995;40(7):1561–8.
3. Uchida K, Masamune A, Shimosegawa T, et al. Prevalence of IgG4-related disease in Japan based on nationwide survey in 2009. Int J Rheumatol 2012; 2012:358371.
4. Weber SM, Cubukcu-Dimopulo O, Palesty JA, et al. Lymphoplasmacytic sclerosing pancreatitis: inflammatory mimic of pancreatic carcinoma. J Gastrointest Surg 2003;7(1):129–37 [discussion: 137–9].
5. Hardacre JM, Iacobuzio-Donahue CA, Sohn TA, et al. Results of pancreaticoduodenectomy for lymphoplasmacytic sclerosing pancreatitis. Ann Surg 2003; 237(6):853–8 [discussion: 858–9].
6. Hamano H, Kawa S, Horiuchi A, et al. High serum IgG4 concentrations in patients with sclerosing pancreatitis. N Engl J Med 2001;344(10):732–8.
7. Shimosegawa T, Chari ST, Frulloni L, et al. International Consensus Diagnostic Criteria for autoimmune pancreatitis: guidelines of the International Association of Pancreatology. Pancreas 2011;40(3):352–8.
8. Kamisawa T, Chari ST, Giday SA, et al. Clinical profile of autoimmune pancreatitis and its histological subtypes: an international multicenter survey. Pancreas 2011; 40(6):809–14.
9. Ghazale A, Chari ST, Zhang L, et al. Immunoglobulin G4-associated cholangitis: clinical profile and response to therapy. Gastroenterology 2008;134(3):706–15.
10. Sah RP, Chari ST, Pannala R, et al. Differences in clinical profile and relapse rate of type 1 versus type 2 autoimmune pancreatitis. Gastroenterology 2010;139(1): 140–8 [quiz: e12–3].
11. Okazaki K, Kawa S, Kamisawa T, et al. Clinical diagnostic criteria of autoimmune pancreatitis: revised proposal. J Gastroenterol 2006;41(7):626–31.
12. Maruyama M, Watanabe T, Kanai K, et al. International Consensus Diagnostic Criteria for autoimmune pancreatitis and its Japanese amendment have improved diagnostic ability over existing criteria. Gastroenterol Res Pract 2013; 2013:456965.
13. Kim KP, Kim MH, Kim JC, et al. Diagnostic criteria for autoimmune chronic pancreatitis revisited. World J Gastroenterol 2006;12(16):2487–96.
14. Otsuki M, Chung JB, Okazaki K, et al. Asian diagnostic criteria for autoimmune pancreatitis: consensus of the Japan-Korea Symposium on Autoimmune Pancreatitis. J Gastroenterol 2008;43(6):403–8.
15. Chari ST, Smyrk TC, Levy MJ, et al. Diagnosis of autoimmune pancreatitis: the Mayo Clinic experience. Clin Gastroenterol Hepatol 2006;4(8):1010–6.
16. Raina A, Yadav D, Krasinskas AM, et al. Evaluation and management of autoimmune pancreatitis: experience at a large US center. Am J Gastroenterol 2009; 104(9):2295–306.
17. Farrell JJ, Garber J, Sahani D, et al. EUS findings in patients with autoimmune pancreatitis. Gastrointest Endosc 2004;60(6):927–36.
18. Numata K, Ozawa Y, Kobayashi N, et al. Contrast-enhanced sonography of autoimmune pancreatitis: comparison with pathologic findings. J Ultrasound Med 2004;23(2):199–206.
19. Zaheer A, Singh VK, Akshintala VS, et al. Differentiating autoimmune pancreatitis from pancreatic adenocarcinoma using dual-phase computed tomography. J Comput Assist Tomogr 2014;38(1):146–52.
20. Takahashi N, Fletcher JG, Hough DM, et al. Autoimmune pancreatitis: differentiation from pancreatic carcinoma and normal pancreas on the basis of

enhancement characteristics at dual-phase CT. AJR Am J Roentgenol 2009; 193(2):479–84.

21. Lee-Felker SA, Felker ER, Kadell B, et al. Use of MDCT to differentiate autoimmune pancreatitis from ductal adenocarcinoma and interstitial pancreatitis. AJR Am J Roentgenol 2015;205(1):2–9.

22. Sugumar A, Levy MJ, Kamisawa T, et al. Endoscopic retrograde pancreatography criteria to diagnose autoimmune pancreatitis: an international multicentre study. Gut 2011;60(5):666–70.

23. Ghazale A, Chari ST, Smyrk TC, et al. Value of serum IgG4 in the diagnosis of autoimmune pancreatitis and in distinguishing it from pancreatic cancer. Am J Gastroenterol 2007;102(8):1646–53.

24. Frulloni L, Lunardi C, Simone R, et al. Identification of a novel antibody associated with autoimmune pancreatitis. N Engl J Med 2009;361(22):2135–42.

25. Kino-Ohsaki J, Nishimori I, Morita M, et al. Serum antibodies to carbonic anhydrase I and II in patients with idiopathic chronic pancreatitis and Sjogren's syndrome. Gastroenterology 1996;110(5):1579–86.

26. Kim KP, Kim MH, Song MH, et al. Autoimmune chronic pancreatitis. Am J Gastroenterol 2004;99(8):1605–16.

27. Ralli S, Lin J, Farrell J. Autoimmune pancreatitis. N Engl J Med 2007;356(15): 1586 [author reply: 1587].

28. Hamano H, Arakura N, Muraki T, et al. Prevalence and distribution of extrapancreatic lesions complicating autoimmune pancreatitis. J Gastroenterol 2006;41(12): 1197–205.

29. Nishino T, Toki F, Oyama H, et al. Biliary tract involvement in autoimmune pancreatitis. Pancreas 2005;30(1):76–82.

30. Nakazawa T, Ohara H, Sano H, et al. Cholangiography can discriminate sclerosing cholangitis with autoimmune pancreatitis from primary sclerosing cholangitis. Gastrointest Endosc 2004;60(6):937–44.

31. Nakazawa T, Ohara H, Sano H, et al. Clinical differences between primary sclerosing cholangitis and sclerosing cholangitis with autoimmune pancreatitis. Pancreas 2005;30(1):20–5.

32. Wang WL, Farris AB, Lauwers GY, et al. Autoimmune pancreatitis-related cholecystitis: a morphologically and immunologically distinctive form of lymphoplasmacytic sclerosing cholecystitis. Histopathology 2009;54(7):829–36.

33. Sumimoto K, Uchida K, Mitsuyama T, et al. A proposal of a diagnostic algorithm with validation of International Consensus Diagnostic Criteria for autoimmune pancreatitis in a Japanese cohort. Pancreatology 2013;13(3):230–7.

34. Levy MJ, Reddy RP, Wiersema MJ, et al. EUS-guided Trucut biopsy in establishing autoimmune pancreatitis as the cause of obstructive jaundice. Gastrointest Endosc Mar 2005;61(3):467–72.

35. Iwashita T, Yasuda I, Doi S, et al. Use of samples from endoscopic ultrasound-guided 19-gauge fine-needle aspiration in diagnosis of autoimmune pancreatitis. Clin Gastroenterol Hepatol 2012;10(3):316–22.

36. Kanno A, Ishida K, Hamada S, et al. Diagnosis of autoimmune pancreatitis by EUS-FNA by using a 22-gauge needle based on the International Consensus Diagnostic Criteria. Gastrointest Endosc 2012;76(3):594–602.

37. Deheragoda MG, Church NI, Rodriguez-Justo M, et al. The use of immunoglobulin g4 immunostaining in diagnosing pancreatic and extrapancreatic involvement in autoimmune pancreatitis. Clin Gastroenterol Hepatol 2007;5(10):1229–34.

38. Moon SH, Kim MH, Park DH, et al. Is a 2-week steroid trial after initial negative investigation for malignancy useful in differentiating autoimmune pancreatitis

from pancreatic cancer? A prospective outcome study. Gut 2008;57(12): 1704–12.

39. Hirano K, Tada M, Isayama H, et al. Long-term prognosis of autoimmune pancreatitis with and without corticosteroid treatment. Gut Dec 2007;56(12):1719–24.
40. Kamisawa T, Shimosegawa T, Okazaki K, et al. Standard steroid treatment for autoimmune pancreatitis. Gut 2009;58(11):1504–7.
41. Buijs J, van Heerde MJ, Rauws EA, et al. Comparable efficacy of low- versus high-dose induction corticosteroid treatment in autoimmune pancreatitis. Pancreas 2014;43(2):261–7.
42. Hart PA, Kamisawa T, Brugge WR, et al. Long-term outcomes of autoimmune pancreatitis: a multicentre, international analysis. Gut 2013;62(12):1771–6.
43. Maire F, Le Baleur Y, Rebours V, et al. Outcome of patients with type 1 or 2 autoimmune pancreatitis. Am J Gastroenterol 2011;106(1):151–6.
44. Rueda JC, Duarte-Rey C, Casas N. Successful treatment of relapsing autoimmune pancreatitis in primary Sjogren's syndrome with rituximab: report of a case and review of the literature. Rheumatol Int 2009;29(12):1481–5.
45. Sandanayake NS, Church NI, Chapman MH, et al. Presentation and management of post-treatment relapse in autoimmune pancreatitis/immunoglobulin G4-associated cholangitis. Clin Gastroenterol Hepatol 2009;7(10):1089–96.
46. Hart PA, Topazian MD, Witzig TE, et al. Treatment of relapsing autoimmune pancreatitis with immunomodulators and rituximab: the Mayo Clinic experience. Gut 2013;62(11):1607–15.
47. Topazian M, Witzig TE, Smyrk TC, et al. Rituximab therapy for refractory biliary strictures in immunoglobulin G4-associated cholangitis. Clin Gastroenterol Hepatol 2008;6(3):364–6.

The Role of Endoscopic Retrograde Cholangiopancreatography in Management of Pancreatic Diseases

Brian P. Riff, MD[a], Vinay Chandrasekhara, MD[b],*

KEYWORDS

- Acute pancreatitis • Autoimmune pancreatitis • Chronic pancreatitis
- Pancreatic divisum • Pancreatic duct leaks • Pancreatic duct strictures
- Sphincter of Oddi dysfunction • Pancreatic cancer

KEY POINTS

- Endoscopic retrograde cholangiopancreatography is an effective platform for a variety of therapies in the management of benign and malignant disease of the pancreas.
- Over the last 50 years, endotherapy has evolved into the first-line therapy in the majority of acute and chronic inflammatory diseases of the pancreas.
- Gastroenterologists must maintain knowledge of procedure indication and sufficient procedure volume to handle complex pancreatic endotherapy.

BACKGROUND

Endoscopic retrograde cholangiopancreatography (ERCP) was first described in 1968 as a diagnostic tool for evaluating disorders of the pancreas or biliary tract.[1] Since then, advances in technique and instruments such as endoscopic sphincterotomy, lithotripsy, and stenting have evolved ERCP from a diagnostic test to a therapeutic platform for a variety of interventions.[2–5] The usefulness of ERCP in management of malignant obstruction is well-established.[6] In this article, we discuss the usefulness of endoscopic retrograde pancreatography (ERP) in the management of benign diseases, including acute pancreatitis (AP), recurrent AP (RAP), and chronic pancreatitis

[a] Division of Gastroenterology, Icahn School of Medicine at Mount Sinai, One Gustave L. Levy Place, Box 1069, New York, NY 10029, USA; [b] Division of Gastroenterology, University of Pennsylvania Perelman School of Medicine, 3400 Civic Center Boulevard, Perelman Center for Advanced Medicine South Pavilion, 7th Floor, Philadelphia, PA 19104, USA
* Corresponding author.
E-mail address: vinay.chandrasekhara@uphs.upenn.edu

Gastroenterol Clin N Am 45 (2016) 45–65
http://dx.doi.org/10.1016/j.gtc.2015.10.009
0889-8553/16/$ – see front matter © 2016 Elsevier Inc. All rights reserved.

(CP), as well as pancreatic duct (PD) leaks, fistulas, and fluid collections. In addition, we will address techniques and interventions used for reducing the risk of post-ERCP pancreatitis (PEP).

ACUTE PANCREATITIS

AP is common, with more than 200,000 admissions annually in the United States.[7] The 2 most common etiologies of AP are heavy alcohol consumption and gallstones, which account for up to 80% of AP.[8,9] In up to 20% of cases, no etiology can be identified readily after a thorough history, physical examination, and abdominal imaging.[10] In prospective studies of a single episode of idiopathic AP, endoscopic ultrasonography (EUS) has been shown to reliably identify the cause in up to 79% of cases, with common findings including choledocholithiasis, biliary sludge, CP, or tumor not seen on cross-sectional imaging.[11,12] As such, EUS is recommended in individuals 40 years of age or older with AP and no identifiable etiology.[13,14]

Given the accuracy of EUS and favorable safety profile, ERCP after a single episode of unexplained pancreatitis is generally not recommended.[15] However, there are certain situations, such as gallstone pancreatitis, wherein early ERCP can facilitate an endoscopic intervention in AP that has favorable outcomes.

Gallstone Pancreatitis

Gallstone pancreatitis accounts for between 35% and 60% of all cases of AP.[16] Most cases are typically self-limiting, but up to 25% of cases can be severe with associated end-organ dysfunction and death, with a mortality rate between 5% and 10%.[17,18] An increase in the alanine aminotransferase of greater than 3 times the upper limit of normal has a positive predictive value of gallstone pancreatitis of 95%.[19] The exact mechanism by which passage of gallstones results in pancreatitis is unknown. One theory proposes that the pathophysiology of gallstone pancreatitis occurs in 2 phases. The first phase is the passage of a small gallstone through the distal duct, initiating the attack of AP. A patent ampulla allows for flow of pancreatic digestive enzymes and a mild attack. In the second phase, additional stones pass through the duct or a stone becomes lodged in the distal duct resulting in either a transient or a continuous obstruction in the common bile duct and PD. The obstruction prevents outflow of activated pancreatic enzymes, PD hypertension, and increased pancreatic enzyme activation.[20] Prior studies have shown an increased incidence of retained stones in severe forms of gallstone pancreatitis compared with mild cases, which forms the theoretic basis for ERCP in AP.[21]

Data on the optimal management of suspected choledocholithiasis in patients with acute biliary pancreatitis are conflicting. Numerous trials have investigated the role of early ERCP (within 72 hours of admission) with or without sphincterotomy compared with conservative management with disparate results.[22–27] Some studies indicated a benefit for early ERCP, whereas others had worse outcomes compared with conservative management. Given the heterogeneity of these studies, multiple metaanalyses and systematic reviews on this topic have been conducted with different inclusion criteria and, therefore, have arrived at different conclusions.[28–32] Many of the original studies included a high percentage of patients who underwent ERCP without identification of any common bile duct stone.[25] In addition, one of the key confounders in this literature is the presence of cholangitis, which has clear data to support the use of early ERCP for decompression.[33]

The most recent metaanalysis on this subject, which specifically excluded cholangitis, showed no significant benefit for early ERCP with or without sphincterotomy on morbidity (relative risk [RR], 0.82; 95% CI, 0.64–1.04) or mortality (RR, 1.22; 95% CI, 0.61–2.45), regardless of the predicted severity of gallstone pancreatitis.[29] Another review with slightly different inclusion criteria had a similar finding that early ERCP in the absence of cholangitis was associated with a nonsignificant reduction in overall complications (RR, 0.76; 95% CI, 0.41–1.04) but a nonsignificant increase in mortality (RR, 1.13; 95% CI, 0.23–5.63).[28] If a patient has evidence of cholangitis with AP, early ERCP reduces mortality significantly (RR, 0.20; 95% CI, 0.06–0.68) as well as local and systemic complications (RR, 0.45; 95% CI, 0.20–0.99). Similarly, if a patient has evidence of biliary obstruction (conjugated bilirubin of >2 mg/dL and common bile duct dilation of >6 mm, gallbladder in situ) and AP, early ERCP significantly reduced local and systemic complications (RR, 0.54; 95% CI, 0.32–0.91). Given these findings, ERCP should only be performed in the setting of AP with coexisting cholangitis or persistent biliary obstruction.[32,34]

Post–Endoscopic Retrograde Cholangiopancreatography Pancreatitis

Pancreatitis is the most common serious adverse event associated with ERCP with an incidence of 3% to 10% in most large series.[35,36] Certain patient and procedure-related recognized risk factors are associated with a higher incidence of PEP (**Box 1**).

The administration of rectal indomethacin and certain procedural techniques such as wire-guided access and pancreatic stent placement, can mitigate the risk of PEP.[37–39] Trauma-induced papillary edema can lead to pancreatic sphincter obstruction and resultant ductal hypertension. It is thought that, by immediately placing a PD stent, the pressure gradient is decreased across the pancreatic sphincter and the risk for PEP is also decreased. In patients who are perceived to be at high risk for PEP,

---

Box 1
Risk Factors for PEP

Patient-related Risk Factors

Prior PEP

Suspected SOD

Previous recurrent acute pancreatitis

Female gender

Younger age

Normal serum bilirubin

Absence of pancreatic mass or chronic pancreatitis

Procedure-related Risk Factors

Difficult cannulation

Pancreatic sphincterotomy

Contrast injection into the pancreatic duct

Biliary sphincter balloon dilation of an intact sphincter

Abbreviations: PEP, post endoscopic retrograde pancreatography pancreatitis; SOD, Sphincter of Oddi dysfunction.
Data from Freeman ML, DiSario JA, Nelson DB, et al. Risk factors for post-ERCP pancreatitis: a prospective, multicenter study. Gastrointest Endosc 2001;54(4):425–34; and Choudhary A, Bechtold ML, Arif M, et al. Pancreatic stents for prophylaxis against post-ERCP pancreatitis: a meta-analysis and systematic review. Gastrointest Endosc 2011;73(2):275–82.

prophylactic pancreatic stent placement decreases the risk of pancreatitis (15.5% vs 5.8%). This reduction translates to a number needed to stent of only 10 to prevent 1 episode of PEP.[37] In a recent metaanalysis (n = 1422), the administration of rectal indomethacin near the time of ERCP reduced the risk of PEP (odds ratio [OR], 0.49; 95% CI, 0.34–0.71; $P<.01$) as compared with placebo.[40] The timing of administration has varied in multiple studies including 2 hours before, immediately before, during, and immediately after ERCP with similar results. There is ongoing research to evaluate whether the administration of indomethacin alone is sufficient to protect against PEP; however, currently, the administration of indomethacin (100 mg per rectum administered periprocedurally) in addition to placement of a PD stent is suggested for prevention of PEP in high-risk patients. At this time, the European Society of Gastrointestinal Endoscopy and American College of Gastroenterology guidelines state that rectal nonsteroidal anti-inflammatory drugs, if available, should be considered in preventing PEP in high-risk individuals.[13,41]

RECURRENT ACUTE PANCREATITIS

RAP is defined as the occurrence of 2 or more episodes of AP in a patient without any evidence of CP.[42] In a patient with an initial episode of AP, the lifetime risk of RAP is 17% to 20%.[43] Much like AP, the most common etiologies of RAP include heavy alcohol use and gallstones. The etiology of RAP can be identified in the majority of patients. Other common etiologies include anatomic variants such as pancreas divisum or aberrant pancreatobiliary junction, sphincter of Oddi dysfunction (SOD), hereditary etiologies (CFTR, PRSS1, SPINK1), and metabolic conditions such as hypercalcemia and hypertriglyceridemia. A thorough history and physical examination in conjunction with a complete metabolic panel, transabdominal ultrasonography, MR cholangiopancreatography (MRCP), and computed tomography (CT) scan detect the cause of RAP in 70% of cases.[44]

Pancreas Divisum

Pancreas divisum is a congenital variant in the anatomy of the PD system. The ventral and dorsal PDs fail to fuse during organogenesis and the majority of the pancreas is drained via the dorsal duct into the minor papilla. This variant is relatively common and present in 2% to 10% of the population in autopsy studies.[45] Although most patients with this ductal variant are asymptomatic throughout life, there is a small subset (approximately 5% of patients with divisum) that develops AP and/or chronic abdominal pain.[46] Although pancreas divisum is often present in individuals with idiopathic AP, the role of divisum as a cause of RAP or CP is controversial.[47–49] The presence of divisum does not automatically implicate that as the cause of AP or CP. The putative hypothesis is that the caliber of the minor papilla is too narrow to drain the pancreatic secretions via the dorsal duct creating a relative outflow obstruction as seen on secretin stimulated MRI studies leading to pain and possibly acute or CP or increased risk of pancreatitis from accepted stimuli such as alcohol or CFTR mutations.[50,51]

The gold standard for diagnosis of divisum is ERP. Contrast injection into the ventral duct through the major papilla shows a short duct tapering terminally into side branches within the pancreatic head, whereas injection through the minor papilla demonstrates a patent dorsal system draining the pancreatic body and tail (**Fig. 1**).[52] However, this modality is not the favored diagnostic test for divisum owing to a significantly higher rate of post-PEP with dorsal duct cannulation (OR, 7.45; 95% CI, 3.25–17.07).[53] As such, alternative diagnostic tests are preferred to establish the

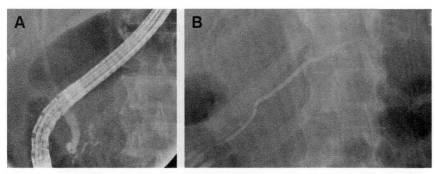

Fig. 1. Pancreatogram demonstrating pancreas divisum. (*A*) Ventral duct injection demonstrating a short duct with terminal side branches. (*B*) Contrast injection through the minor papilla demonstrates a dominant dorsal duct.

presence of divisum, including EUS, CT, and MRI. In a retrospective review of all patients who had a diagnosis of pancreas divisum confirmed on ERP, the sensitivity of EUS for pancreas divisum was 86.7%, significantly higher than sensitivity for CT (15.5%) or MRCP (60%).[54] An infusion of secretin before MRCP (secretin-enhanced MRCP) significantly increases the sensitivity (84.5 vs 74.2; $P = .02$) and specificity (88.1 vs 76.2; $P = .01$) of diagnosing pancreas divisum compared with traditional MRCP.[55]

Much like the causal relationship between pancreas divisum and pancreatitis, the usefulness of endotherapy in preventing recurrent pancreatitis or improving abdominal symptoms in patients with identified pancreas divisum is an area of debate. The goal of endotherapy is to enlarge the orifice of the minor papilla through papillotomy or stenting to relieve the presumed obstruction of pancreatic exocrine flow. One of the original studies was a small clinical trial of patients with pancreas divisum and at least 2 prior documented episodes of pancreatitis. Patients were randomized to either ERP via the minor papilla with dorsal duct stenting versus no intervention. Over a follow-up period of 30 months, the stenting group had significant fewer hospitalizations, documented episodes of pancreatitis, and baseline episodes of abdominal pain.[56] Many larger studies have been conducted since that time with promising results on preventing RAP but limited benefit in the treatment of chronic pain. A retrospective evaluation of 24 patients with divisum and RAP without CP were treated with either minor papilla sphincterotomy or dorsal duct stenting and followed for a median of 39 months (range, 24–105). There was a significant decrease in recurrent episodes of pancreatitis, but no benefit in baseline pain control.[57] Results of endotherapy in patients with evidence of CP and divisum in preventing RAP seem less promising. In a retrospective study of 113 patients who had undergone endotherapy for divisum, primary success defined as either a clinical improvement or cure was noted to be 53.2% in RAP patients, but only 18.2% patients with features of CP. On multivariate analysis, younger age (46.5 vs 58; $P<.0001$) and CP (OR, 0.10; 95% CI, 0.03–0.39) were independent predictors of failed response to endotherapy.[58] A recent metaanalysis on this subject included 838 patients from 22 studies. Patients with RAP had a response rate ranging from 43% to 100% (median, 76%). Response rates were lower for patients with CP (21%–80%; median, 42%) and chronic abdominal pain (11%–55%; median, 33%).[59] Given these findings, it seems reasonable to suggest endotherapy for patients with divisum who have clearly documented episodes of RAP without another obvious etiology. Because these patients are at increased risk for PEP, administration of rectal indomethacin is recommended to reduce that risk.[60] Routine endotherapy in patients with CP and/or chronic abdominal pain in the presence of pancreas divisum is not recommended, and needs to be individualized on a case-by-case basis.

Sphincter of Oddi Dysfunction

SOD is a heterogeneous group of clinical syndromes. Biliary SOD typically presents as biliary type pain, and is often seen in patients after cholecystectomy, whereas pancreatic SOD is associated with idiopathic recurrent pancreatitis.

The revised Milwaukee Biliary Group classification has been used to diagnose, categorize, and drive intervention in suspected SOD patients. Type I biliary SOD consists of patients with biliary-type pain, abnormal aminotransferases, bilirubin or alkaline phosphatase (>2 times normal values) documented on 2 or more occasions, and a dilated bile duct (>8 mm on ultrasound). Approximately 65% to 95% of these patients have manometric evidence of biliary SOD. Type II patients present with biliary-type pain and one of the laboratory or imaging abnormalities mentioned. Approximately 50% to 63% of these patients have manometric evidence of biliary SOD. Type III patients present with recurrent biliary-type pain without any other findings. Approximately 12% to 59% of these patients have manometric evidence of biliary SOD.

Management of type I SOD is accepted to be ERCP with biliary sphincterotomy without the need for sphincter of Oddi manometry (SOM).[61] Type II SOD has less objective evidence of a fixed abnormality compared with type I. It is recommended that all patients with suspected type II SOD undergo ERCP with SOM-directed sphincterotomy or empiric biliary with or without pancreatic sphincterotomy.[14] The recommendation for SOM in patients with suspected type II SOD is based on 2 prior randomized clinical trials, the largest of which included 47 patients.[62,63] All patients underwent SOM and then were randomized to either a true biliary sphincterotomy or a sham sphincterotomy. At 1-year follow-up, there was a significant improvement in pain in patients who had undergone sphincterotomy (65% vs 30%; P<.01), which was best predicted by a SOM basal pressure of greater than 40 mm Hg. Patients in the sham sphincterotomy were crossed over to open-label sphincterotomy and again an elevated basal pressure was predictive of a response to endotherapy.[62] Conversely, large retrospective or nonrandomized trials have shown that the result of SOM is less predictive of response to sphincterotomy. Three trials where sphincterotomy was performed in all patients with suspected type II SOD had a good clinical response (47%–100%) without any correlation to SOM.[64–66] Other studies have shown a good pain response to empiric sphincterotomy without performance of SOM or need for pancreatography.[67] It is because of this unclear relationship between manometric findings, disease etiology, and response to therapy that the American Society for Gastrointestinal Endoscopy and experts in the field acknowledge that ERCP with empiric biliary sphincterotomy is an alternative to SOM-guided therapy.[14,61,68]

The recently conducted EPISOD (Evaluating Predictors and Interventions in Sphincter of Oddi Dysfunction) trial may have been the definitive study to show that there is no role for endotherapy in individuals with type III SOD.[69] In this multicenter, sham-controlled, randomized clinical trial, 214 patients with typical biliary type pain after cholecystectomy without laboratory abnormality or biliary dilation were randomized to sphincterotomy or sham regardless of SOM findings. Patients with increased pancreatic sphincter pressures on SOM who were randomized to the sphincterotomy arm were then randomized again to biliary or both a biliary and pancreatic sphincterotomy. There was a significant improvement in pain in the sham group compared with the sphincterotomy group (37% vs 23%; $P = .01$). In addition to not providing any relief of pain, there was a 12% rate of PEP despite the placement of a PD stent in all patients. Based on these results, patients with type III SOD should not be offered ERCP or sphincterotomy.[70]

Although biliary SOD is associated with a specific pain syndrome and risk for PEP, pancreatic SOD is thought to be a risk factor for RAP. In patients previously diagnosed with idiopathic RAP, manometric evidence of SOD is considered to be a risk factor for a future episode of pancreatitis (hazard ratio, 4.3; 95% CI, 1.3–14.5; $P<.02$).[71]

Like biliary SOD, pancreatic SOD has 3 subtypes. Type I refers to patients with typical pancreatic type pain with an increased serum amylase or lipase more than 1.5 to 2 times the upper limit of normal on 2 separate occasions and pancreatic ductal dilation ($\geq$6 mm in the head and $\geq$5 mm in the body). Type II includes patients with pancreatic type pain with either increased pancreatic enzyme levels or ductal dilation. Finally, type III refers to patients with pancreatic type pain in the absence of laboratory or radiographic abnormalities.[72,73]

In patients who have RAP and manometrically confirmed SOD, sphincterotomy has been effective in reducing the rate of recurrent pancreatitis and improving pancreatic type pain.[74,75] Although these studies were statistically significant in reducing the rate and frequency of AP, the rate of at least 1 recurrent episode of pancreatitis in patients who had undergone sphincterotomy was still 51% at 11 years of follow-up.[74] Of note, the rate of recurrent pancreatitis was not different in patients who underwent biliary sphincterotomy (51.5%) versus dual biliary and pancreatic sphincterotomy (52.8%).[71] As such, pancreatic sphincterotomy should not be pursued in this patient population given the independent risks associated with this procedure.[76]

CHRONIC PANCREATITIS

CP is an irreversible inflammatory process leading to fibrotic changes with destruction of the pancreatic parenchyma with impairment of the exocrine and endocrine function. Based on morphology, CP can be classified as a large duct type and a small duct type, both of which can occur with or without calcifications. ERP can play 2 major roles in CP: diagnostic in the setting of uncertainty and therapeutic ductal drainage in the setting of large duct disease. The goal of main pancreatic duct (MPD) drainage is relief of ductal hypertension and subsequent pain control.

ERP is sensitive for identifying ductal changes in CP, but cannot assess for parenchymal changes and is thus insensitive for evaluating for minimal change disease.[77] The Cambridge classification of pancreatography findings is the traditional system to identify patients with CP and grade severity. The classification is based on changes in the MPD including dilation, strictures, and irregular contour, as well as the number of irregular side branches plus miscellaneous features, such as filling defects in the MPD or filling cavities.[78] As it turns out, these findings have poor sensitivity and specificity. The results are operator dependent with respect to both interpretation of the pancreatogram, and performance of an adequate contrast injection to ensure proper duct filling. In addition, findings that are classified as CP by the Cambridge classification can also be seen in older patients or in patients who drink alcohol without any other clinical or radiographic features of CP.[79–81] Most important, pancreatography cannot assess properly parenchymal changes that are the primary finding in minimal change CP. In some cases of CP, no obvious changes are noted on imaging and the diagnosis is made on a basis of exocrine insufficiency. It is for this reason that other diagnostic tests are preferred to establish the diagnosis of CP, with ERP typically reserved for therapy.

Pancreatic endotherapy may be effective in relieving pain in individuals with uncomplicated chronic calcific pancreatitis and should be considered as the first line therapy for ductal decompression. It can be achieved by performing pancreatic sphincterotomy, stricture management with dilating and placement of pancreatic stents, and stone lithotripsy. Clinical response should be evaluated at 6 to 8 weeks. If there is no improvement in subjective measurements of pain or objective improvements in weight, diarrhea, or nutrition, then surgical decompression should be pursued.[14,82,83] In a randomized clinical trial comparing endoscopic and surgical drainage of the MPD, surgery had significant improvement in pain (75% vs 32%; P = .007) and heath summary scores. Rates of complication, duration of hospital stay, and changes in pancreatic function were similar between the 2 groups.[84] This study only enrolled 39 patients in total and many experts feel that surgical intervention carries increased risks relative to endoscopic therapy. Regardless of the modality, smoking and alcohol cessation should be part of the treatment recommendations.[85]

Pancreatic Duct Strictures

In a large, multicenter study of endoscopic therapy in CP, MPD obstruction was caused by strictures (47%), stones (18%), or a combination of both (32%).[86] MPD strictures may be single or multifocal. Most strictures occur in the pancreatic head caused by inflammation or fibrosis. A dominant stricture is defined as having at least one of the following characteristics: upstream MPD dilation 6 mm or greater in diameter or prevention of contrast outflow along a 6-Fr catheter inserted upstream from the stricture.[87] The presence of multiple or tail strictures is the main predictor of pain recurrence.[88,89]

CP is associated with an increased risk of pancreatic cancer. Approximately 2% of patients with a new diagnosis of CP have an underlying pancreatic malignancy.[90] As such, MPD strictures must be evaluated carefully using contrast-enhanced cross-sectional imaging such as a pancreas protocol CT. In addition, consideration should be given to assessment of tumor markers and extensive sample collection, including EUS-guided fine needle aspiration of suspicious areas.[91]

The goal of endotherapy in PD strictures is remediation of the strictures to allow pancreatic drainage. These strictures tend to be very tight and require serial dilation and stent placement. The first part of stricture management is performing a pancreatic sphincterotomy. Unlike biliary stenting, a pancreatic sphincterotomy was performed before MPD stenting in all major trials and is recommended by the European Society of Gastrointestinal Endoscopy.[82] A short, 5- to 6-mm pancreatic sphincterotomy is performed with the cutting wire oriented to the 1 to 2 o'clock position with the very distal part of the cutting wire.[92] An isolated pancreatic sphincterotomy is not associated with an increased risk for biliary stenosis and thus a concomitant biliary sphincterotomy is not necessary.[93] Once the pancreatic sphincterotomy is performed, attention is paid to stricture management. The standard of care is to perform dilation followed by stent placement. Dilation alone is typically not effective and not recommended. The size of the stent should be chosen to be at least as large as the PD and traverse the stenosis but short enough to minimize ductal changes. A 10-Fr plastic stent has been associated with a decreased hospital admission rate when compared with other smaller stent sizes.[94]

Alternatively, other trials have used multiple, smaller caliber plastic stents to avoid blockage of side branches.[95,96] There have been no trials comparing the efficacy of a single large plastic stent versus multiple smaller stents. Pancreatic stents are prone to occlusion in this indication and stent exchange should be planned every 3 to 6 months for an expected total duration of 12 to 24 months. There have been limited number of case series using fully covered self-expanding metal stents (SEMS) with management of MPD strictures with good efficacy; however, the data are too sparse to recommend this approach at this time.[82,97]

Criteria for definitively removing the stent consists of adequate outflow of contrast medium into the duodenum within 1 to 2 minutes after ductal filling upstream from the dilated stricture immediately after stent removal plus extraction of ductal debris, and easy passage of a 6-Fr catheter through the dilated stricture.[98,99] The size of the MPD after the stenting protocol is not predictive of pain recurrence even in the presence of a persistent stricture.[95,100]

Regardless of the size and length of stent chosen, endoscopic therapy with dilation and stenting for MPD strictures without intraductal stones has been effective in decreasing abdominal pain in 65% to 84% of patients.[99,101] After definitive stent removal, 27% to 38% of patients will relapse with pain at a median of 25 months. With a pain relapse, patients should be offered restenting. Long-term follow-up of MPD stenting shows similar efficacy with satisfactory pain control in 52% to 90% of patients when followed out to 6 years with fewer than 30% of patients ultimately needing surgical decompression.[100,102,103]

Complications of MPD stenting can occur. Stent occlusion was the most common (65% at 3 months in 1 study), and is the reason for the planned stent exchanges a priori.[95] Stent migration occurred in 10% of the study patients.[104] Stent migration can be distal with impaction on the opposite wall of the duodenum and rarely results in perforation. Alternatively, proximal migration, which can be technically challenging to manage, particularly in the presence of a high-grade stricture, can occur into the pancreas. Careful selection of stents such as those with side wings and pigtail stents can decrease the risk of migration.[105]

Pancreatic Duct Stones

Similar to MPD strictures, PD calculi are a common complication of CP and produce pain by causing upstream dilation and ductal hypertension (**Fig. 2**). PD stones are seen in approximately 50% of patients with CP.[86] Stones less than 5 mm in size without any

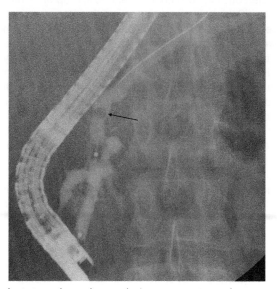

Fig. 2. Pancreatic duct stone (*arrow*) seen during pancreatography.

evidence of an MPD stricture can typically be removed by a Dormia basket or an extraction balloon after a pancreatic sphincterotomy.[106] Complete or partial pain relief after pancreatic sphincterotomy and mechanical stone extraction is seen in 50% to 77%.[107,108] However, in cases of stones greater than 5 mm in diameter, which is larger than the MPD size, located upstream of MPD stricture or impacted in the head of the pancreas, standard extraction techniques are typically ineffective.[109] In these cases stone fragmentation with extracorporeal shock wave lithotripsy (ESWL) is helpful and considered first-line therapy.[82,89,110–113]

The aim of ESWL is to fragment calculi in the MPD to less than 3 mm in size. Multiple metaanalyses have demonstrated the efficacy of ESWL for ductal clearance and pain control. An analysis of 17 studies with a total of 491 patients revealed a clearance rate between 37% to 100% and good pain relief.[114] Another review of 11 studies with more than 1100 patients showed successful stone fragmentation in 89% of patients.[91] A large, single-center study of 1006 patients demonstrated complete pain relief in 42% of patients in 24 to 36 months of follow-up. Only 5% of patients had persistent severe pain.[113]

ESWL therapy is typically offered to patients with large calculi in the head or body and pain as their main complaint. Relative contraindications are patients with isolated calculi in the tail, multiple MPD strictures, mass in the head of the pancreas, pseudocysts or walled off pancreatic necrosis, and pregnancy. Epidural anesthesia is preferred if available.[115] Recurrence of stones is seen in 23% of patients after more than 60 months of follow-up.[113] Minor side effects such as pain and bruising of skin at the site of shock delivery have been described, as well as more serious complications such as pancreatitis, sepsis, and gastric submucosal hematoma.[83]

A comparison of multimodality therapy with ESWL in combination with MPD stenting versus ESWL alone in patients with CP and PD stones demonstrated that pain relapse at 2 years was similar in both groups (45% vs 38%; $P = .63$); however, the cost of the additional endotherapy added almost 3 times the cost.[111] The addition of ESWL to endoscopic stenting and stone clearance has been shown to be effective. One study of 120 patients demonstrated partial pain relief in 85% and complete pain relief requiring no narcotics in 50% after a mean follow-up of 51 months.[116] As such, the current American Society for Gastrointestinal Endoscopy guidelines recommend that ESWL be used as an adjunct for patients with symptoms attributed to pancreaticolithiasis who are refractory to standard ERCP stone extraction techniques.[14]

Intraductal lithotripsy using laser or electrohydraulic lithotripsy through direct pancreatoscopy is only recommended as second line management if ESWL is not effective or available.[117] Despite that, per oral pancreatoscopy is attractive because it allows for intraductal lithotripsy during the same session as stricture management via ERCP. A large, retrospective study of 46 patients treated over 11 years for PD stones using per oral pancreatoscopy–directed laser or electrohydraulic lithotripsy had a clinical success of complete stone clearance in 74% of patients after a median of 2 ERCPs. There was no difference in efficacy between patients treated with laser or electrohydraulic lithotripsy.[118] Similarly, a multicenter study reported a clinical success of 89% in per oral pancreatoscopy–directed laser lithotripsy for PD stones.[119] The recent introduction of a digital cholangiopancreatoscope is likely to increase this approach compared with ESWL going forward.[120]

Autoimmune Pancreatitis

Autoimmune pancreatitis (AIP) is a distinct form of pancreatitis associated with minimal pain, obstructive jaundice with or without a mass, and hypergammaglobulinemia that readily responds to steroid therapy.[121] There are 2 forms of AIP. Type 1 is the classic disease phenotype more commonly seen in Asia of older males (>80% are males >50 years of age).[122,123] It is associated with a lymphoplasmocytic sclerosing pancreatitis on histology and elevated serum levels immunoglobulin (Ig)G4.[124] In addition to the pancreas, there is often multi-organ involvement in IgG4-associated systemic disease including biliary, eye, kidney, retroperitoneum, and salivary glands.[125] Type 2 AIP is seen in younger patients and is more common in the West. It is a duct-centric pancreatitis with a dense neutrophilic infiltration. Unlike type 1 AIP, serum levels of IgG4 are not increased in type 2. In addition, it is a disease isolated to the pancreas without systemic involvement.[126]

ERP may play an important role in the diagnostic pathway in AIP. The International Consensus Diagnostic Criteria for AIP recommends a pancreatogram be performed when the diagnosis of AIP (type 1 and type 2) is not conclusive based on imaging and laboratory assessment. In addition, if type 2 AIP is suspected, the expert guideline recommends pancreatogram be performed if a core biopsy is not performed or inconclusive.[127] Typical pancreatogram findings in AIP include a long MPD stricture greater than one-third of the length of the duct, or multiple strictures without upstream dilation. Less specific findings include a focal stricture without upstream ductal dilation and side branches arising from a strictured segment. ERP has a reported sensitivity of 44% and specificity of 92%. Interobserver agreement is poor, with endoscopists in Asia outperforming their Western colleagues.[128] In addition to performing a pancreatogram, ampullary biopsies with staining for IgG4 are recommended at the time of ERCP. The biopsies have a sensitivity of 52% to 80% and specificity of 89% to 100% in the diagnosis of type 1 AIP.[129]

PANCREATIC DUCT LEAKS

PD leaks can occur in the setting of AP, CP, trauma, and iatrogenic injury. Pancreatic injury occurs in 55% of all blunt trauma cases and 8% of penetrating abdominal injuries (**Fig. 3**).[130] Disruption can be partial or complete (no visualization of the PD upstream of the leak) and can present as either an internal or an external leaks. The leak can be from the MPD or a side branch. Examples of internal leaks include pseudocyst, walled off pancreatic necrosis, pancreatic ascites, and high amylase pleural effusion. External leaks present as pancreaticocutaneous fistulas and are typically iatrogenic in etiology.[87,131] Disconnected duct syndrome is a specific PD leak with a complete transection of the MPD, resulting in an isolated segment of the tail of the pancreas. This syndrome typically occurs in the setting of severe AP with pancreatic necrosis and can be seen in up to 50% of these patients.[132] Similarly, patients with walled off pancreatic necrosis are ultimately found to have disconnected duct syndrome in 35% to 70% of cases.[133]

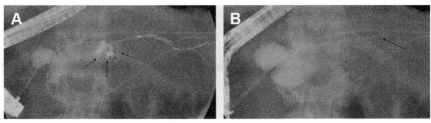

Fig. 3. (*A*) Pancreatogram demonstrating a traumatic pancreatic duct leak (*arrow*) with contrast extravasation. (*B*) A 7-French stent (*arrow*) was placed across the leak.

The clinical presentation of a PD leak is highly variable and, unless overt, the diagnosis depends on having a high degree of suspicion in the appropriate context. Similar to prior discussions, ERP should now only be used in a therapeutic role given the risk of causing or worsening pancreatitis. For internal leaks, a pancreatic protocol CT and MRCP (secretin enhanced if available) are the best initial diagnostic tests.[134] The combination of helical CT and MRCP was 94% accurate in identifying the site of the PD leak.[135] External leaks typically can be diagnosed by fluid analysis for amylase.[136,137]

The management of PD leak depends on the etiology and severity. The majority of PD leaks after pancreatic surgery are low volume and controlled with surgical drains to prevent peritoneal fluid collections, and will spontaneously resolve over days to weeks.[138] Leaks secondary to pancreatitis or trauma often require intervention to resolve in the form of transpapillary drainage. By inserting an endoprosthesis through the major or minor papilla into the MPD, the pressure gradient is altered in favor of pancreatic drainage through the stent rather than the leak. This is also an effective therapy for pancreatic fluid collections that are in direct communication with the PD such as a pseudocyst. In 1 study, the PD leak resolved in 58% of patients treated with transpapillary stenting. On logistic regression, the only factor associated with a successful outcome was bridging the site of the leak with the stent.[139] Multiple other studies have corroborated this finding that bridging the site of the leak is associated with resolution. In addition to bridging, a minimum of 6 weeks of stent placement was associated with successful closure.[140,141]

Transpapillary stenting is successful as a primary therapy for small (<6 cm), communicating pancreatic pseudocysts. Large case series of pseudocysts drained by the transpapillary route have yielded success rates of nearly 90%.[98,140,142] These studies have also shown transpapillary drainage alone is not effective with large pseudocysts (>6 cm) or walled off pancreatic necrosis.[143] In these cases, EUS-guided transmural drainage is the preferred approach. Antibiotic prophylaxis is recommended for endoscopic drainage of sterile pancreatic fluid collections.

PANCREATIC CANCER

ERCP is well-established as a therapeutic platform for biliary decompression in malignancy. The most common cause of malignant biliary obstruction is pancreatic adenocarcinoma followed by cholangiocarcinoma, ampullary neoplasm, and extrinsic compression by portal lymphadenopathy.[144] Up to 70% of patients with pancreatic adenocarcinoma have some degree of biliary obstruction at the time of diagnosis with only 20% of new cases being appropriate for curative resection.[145] The role of ERCP in pancreatobiliary malignancy is biliary decompression for symptom control or as a bridge to surgery in potentially resectable cases. Endoscopic biliary stenting in the setting of a distal malignant obstruction is successful in more than 80% of cases with lower mortality than surgical bypass.[146] In addition to decompression, ERCP can be a diagnostic adjunct in the absence of more sensitive methods such as EUS, although it should not be performed routinely in this setting.

In a randomized clinical trial, preoperative biliary decompression has been to shown to be associated with increased risk of serious complications (39% in the early surgery group vs 74% in the biliary drainage; $P<.001$). There was no mortality benefit or decreased duration of stay in the biliary drainage group.[147] In light of this landmark study and similar retrospective studies, preoperative biliary drainage is not required in the absence of cholangitis or intractable cholestatic symptoms such as pruritus.[148,149] In resectable patients with a compelling indication for decompression, a 10-Fr plastic biliary stent is recommended.

In locally advanced pancreatic cancer, many commonly used neoadjuvant regimens require functioning bilirubin transport mechanisms and bile excretion to avoid toxicity.[150] In this scenario, biliary decompression is indicated. Given a high rate of plastic stent occlusion during neoadjuvant therapy (average patency is 134 days, whereas the average time to surgery is 150 days), the use of a fully covered SEMS has been shown to have decreased occlusion rates and improved outcomes and may be considered as an alternative to plastic stent, recognizing that this is not an indication approved by the US Food and Drug Administration for the device.[151,152]

For unresectable pancreatic malignancy, endoscopic drainage is safer than a surgical biliary bypass (RR of complications 0.6; 95% CI, 0.45–0.81), but with a higher rate of recurrent obstruction.[153] It is for this reason that SEMS are the preferred stent in this indication owing to a superior patency rate when compared with plastic (3.6 vs 1.8 mo; $P<.01$).[154] A metaanalysis of plastic stent versus SEMS in advanced pancreatic cancer showed that SEMS cost 15 to 40 times the cost of plastic stents and are only cost effective if the patient lives 4 months or longer after biliary decompression. One of the studies included showed a median survival time of 2.7 versus 5.3 months with liver metastases. Thus, the authors concluded that SEMS placement is not cost effective in the presence of liver metastases.[155]

SUMMARY

ERCP is an effective platform for a variety of therapies in the management of benign and malignant disease of the pancreas. Over the last 50 years, endotherapy has evolved into first-line therapy in the majority of acute and chronic inflammatory diseases of the pancreas. As this field advances, it is important that gastroenterologists maintain an adequate knowledge of procedure indication, maintain sufficient procedure volume to handle complex pancreatic endotherapy, and understand alternate approaches to pancreatic diseases including medical management, EUS-directed therapy, and surgical options.

REFERENCES

1. McCune WS, Shorb PE, Moscovitz H. Endoscopic cannulation of the ampulla of Vater: a preliminary report. Ann Surg 1968;167(5):752–6.
2. Kawai K, Akasaka Y, Murakami K, et al. Endoscopic sphincterotomy of the ampulla of Vater. Gastrointest Endosc 1974;20(4):148–51.
3. Demling L, Koch H, Classen M, et al. Endoscopic papillotomy and removal of gall-stones: animal experiments and first clinical results (author's transl). Dtsch Med Wochenschr 1974;99(45):2255–7.
4. Koch H, Stolte M, Walz V. Endoscopic lithotripsy in the common bile duct. Endoscopy 1977;9(2):95–8.
5. Zimmon D, Falkenstein D, Clemett A. Endoscopic drains and stents in the biliary tree and pancreas. Gastrointestinal Endoscopy 1980;26(2):81.
6. Andersen JR, Sorensen SM, Kruse A, et al. Randomised trial of endoscopic endoprosthesis versus operative bypass in malignant obstructive jaundice. Gut 1989;30(8):1132–5.
7. Swaroop VS, Chari ST, Clain JE. Severe acute pancreatitis. JAMA 2004;291(23): 2865–8.
8. Frey CF, Zhou H, Harvey DJ, et al. The incidence and case-fatality rates of acute biliary, alcoholic, and idiopathic pancreatitis in California, 1994-2001. Pancreas 2006;33(4):336–44.

9. Whitcomb DC. Acute pancreatitis. N Engl J Med 2006;354(20):2142–50.
10. Wilcox CM, Varadarajulu S, Eloubeidi M. Role of endoscopic evaluation in idiopathic pancreatitis: a systematic review. Gastrointest Endosc 2006;63(7): 1037–45.
11. Yusoff IF, Raymond G, Sahai AV. A prospective comparison of the yield of EUS in primary vs. recurrent idiopathic acute pancreatitis. Gastrointest Endosc 2004; 60(5):673–8.
12. Vila J, Vicuña M, Irisarri R, et al. Diagnostic yield and reliability of endoscopic ultrasonography in patients with idiopathic acute pancreatitis. Scand J Gastroenterol 2010;45(3):375–81.
13. Tenner S, Baillie J, DeWitt J, et al. American College of Gastroenterology guideline: management of acute pancreatitis. Am J Gastroenterol 2013;108(9): 1400–15.
14. Chandrasekhara V, Chathadi KV, Acosta RD, et al. The role of endoscopy in benign pancreatic disease. Gastrointest Endosc 2015;82(2):203–14.
15. Coyle WJ, Pineau BC, Tarnasky PR, et al. Evaluation of unexplained acute and acute recurrent pancreatitis using endoscopic retrograde cholangiopancreatography, sphincter of Oddi manometry and endoscopic ultrasound. Endoscopy 2002;34(8):617–23.
16. Mergener K, Baillie J. Endoscopic treatment for acute biliary pancreatitis: when and in whom? Gastroenterol Clin North Am 1999;28(3):601–13.
17. Frakes JT. Biliary pancreatitis: a review: Emphasizing appropriate endoscopic intervention. J Clin Gastroenterol 1999;28(2):97–109.
18. Toh SK, Phillips S, Johnson CD. A prospective audit against national standards of the presentation and management of acute pancreatitis in the South of England. Gut 2000;46(2):239–43.
19. Tenner S, Dubner H, Steinberg W. Predicting gallstone pancreatitis with laboratory parameters: a meta-analysis. Am J Gastroenterol 1994;89(10):1863–6.
20. Neoptolemos JP. The theory of 'persisting' common bile duct stones in severe gallstone pancreatitis. Ann R Coll Surg Engl 1989;71(5):326–31.
21. Wilson C, Imrie CW, Carter DC. Fatal acute pancreatitis. Gut 1988;29(6):782–8.
22. Neoptolemos J, London N, James D, et al. Controlled trial of urgent endoscopic retrograde cholangiopancreatography and endoscopic sphincterotomy versus conservative treatment for acute pancreatitis due to gallstones. Lancet 1988; 332(8618):979–83.
23. Nowak A, Nowakowska-Dulawa E, Marek T, et al. Final results of the prospective, randomized, controlled study on endoscopic sphincterotomy versus conventional management in acute biliary pancreatitis. Gastroenterology 1995; 108(Suppl A):380.
24. Fölsch UR, Nitsche R, Lüdtke R, et al. Early ERCP and papillotomy compared with conservative treatment for acute biliary pancreatitis. N Engl J Med 1997; 336(4):237–42.
25. Oria A, Cimmino D, Ocampo C, et al. Early endoscopic intervention versus early conservative management in patients with acute gallstone pancreatitis and biliopancreatic obstruction: a randomized clinical trial. Ann Surg 2007;245(1): 10–7.
26. Tang Y, Xu Y, Liao G. Effect of early endoscopic treatment for patients with severe acute biliary pancreatitis. Chin J Gen Surg 2010;19:801–4.
27. Chen P, Hu B, Wang C, et al. Pilot study of urgent endoscopic intervention without fluoroscopy on patients with severe acute biliary pancreatitis in the intensive care unit. Pancreas 2010;39(3):398–402.

28. Petrov MS, van Santvoort HC, Besselink MG, et al. Early endoscopic retrograde cholangiopancreatography versus conservative management in acute biliary pancreatitis without cholangitis: a meta-analysis of randomized trials. Ann Surg 2008;247(2):250–7.
29. Uy MC, Daez M, Sy PP, et al. Early ERCP in acute gallstone pancreatitis without cholangitis: a meta-analysis. JOP 2009;10(3):299–305.
30. Ayub K, Imada R, Slavin J. Endoscopic retrograde cholangiopancreatography in gallstone-associated acute pancreatitis. Cochrane Database Syst Rev 2004;(4):CD003630.
31. Sharma VK, Howden CW. Metaanalysis of randomized controlled trials of endoscopic retrograde cholangiography and endoscopic sphincterotomy for the treatment of acute biliary pancreatitis. Am J Gastroenterol 1999; 94(11):3211–4.
32. Tse F, Yuan Y. Early routine endoscopic retrograde cholangiopancreatography strategy versus early conservative management strategy in acute gallstone pancreatitis. Cochrane Database Syst Rev 2012;(5):CD009779.
33. Lai EC, Mok FP, Tan ES, et al. Endoscopic biliary drainage for severe acute cholangitis. N Engl J Med 1992;326(24):1582–6.
34. Jarcho JA, Fogel EL, Sherman S. ERCP for gallstone pancreatitis. N Engl J Med 2014;370(2):150–7.
35. Freeman ML, Guda NM. Prevention of post-ERCP pancreatitis: a comprehensive review. Gastrointest Endosc 2004;59(7):845–64.
36. Kochar B, Akshintala VS, Afghani E, et al. Incidence, severity, and mortality of post-ERCP pancreatitis: a systematic review by using randomized, controlled trials. Gastrointest Endosc 2015;81(1):143–9.e9.
37. Singh P, Das A, Isenberg G, et al. Does prophylactic pancreatic stent placement reduce the risk of post-ERCP acute pancreatitis? A meta-analysis of controlled trials. Gastrointest Endosc 2004;60(4):544–50.
38. Artifon EL, Sakai P, Cunha JE, et al. Guidewire cannulation reduces risk of post-ERCP pancreatitis and facilitates bile duct cannulation. Am J Gastroenterol 2007;102(10):2147–53.
39. Elmunzer BJ, Scheiman JM, Lehman GA, et al. A randomized trial of rectal indomethacin to prevent post-ERCP pancreatitis. N Engl J Med 2012;366(15): 1414–22.
40. Ahmad D, Lopez KT, Esmadi MA, et al. The effect of indomethacin in the prevention of post-endoscopic retrograde cholangiopancreatography pancreatitis: a meta-analysis. Pancreas 2014;43(3):338–42.
41. Dumonceau JM, Andriulli A, Elmunzer BJ, et al. Prophylaxis of post-ERCP pancreatitis: European Society of Gastrointestinal Endoscopy (ESGE) guideline - updated June 2014. Endoscopy 2014;46(9):799–815.
42. Das R, Yadav D, Papachristou GI. Endoscopic treatment of recurrent acute pancreatitis and smoldering acute pancreatitis. Gastrointest Endosc Clin N Am 2015;25(4):737–48.
43. Lankisch PG, Breuer N, Bruns A, et al. Natural history of acute pancreatitis: a long-term population-based study. Am J Gastroenterol 2009;104(11):2797–805.
44. Testoni PA. Acute recurrent pancreatitis: etiopathogenesis, diagnosis and treatment. World J Gastroenterol 2014;20(45):16891.
45. Agha FP, Williams KD. Pancreas divisum: incidence, detection, and clinical significance. Am J Gastroenterol 1987;82(4):315–20.
46. Burtin P, Person B, Charneau J, et al. Pancreas divisum and pancreatitis: a coincidental association? Endoscopy 1991;23(2):55–8.

47. Cotton PB. Congenital anomaly of pancreas divisum as cause of obstructive pain and pancreatitis. Gut 1980;21(2):105–14.
48. Bernard J, Sahel J, Giovannini M, et al. Pancreas divisum is a probable cause of acute pancreatitis: a report of 137 cases. Pancreas 1990;5(3): 248–54.
49. Richter JM, Schapiro RH, Mulley AG, et al. Association of pancreas divisum and pancreatitis, and its treatment by sphincteroplasty of the accessory ampulla. Gastroenterology 1981;81(6):1104–10.
50. Manfredi R, Costamagna G, Brizi MG, et al. Pancreas divisum and "santorinicele": diagnosis with dynamic MR cholangiopancreatography with secretin stimulation 1. Radiology 2000;217(2):403–8.
51. Bertin C, Pelletier A, Vullierme MP, et al. Pancreas divisum is not a cause of pancreatitis by itself but acts as a partner of genetic mutations. Am J Gastroenterol 2012;107(2):311–7.
52. Klein SD, Affronti JP. Pancreas divisum, an evidence-based review: part I, pathophysiology. Gastrointest Endosc 2004;60(3):419–25.
53. Moffatt DC, Coté GA, Avula H, et al. Risk factors for ERCP-related complications in patients with pancreas divisum: a retrospective study. Gastrointest Endosc 2011;73(5):963–70.
54. Kushnir VM, Wani SB, Fowler K, et al. Sensitivity of endoscopic ultrasound, multidetector computed tomography, and magnetic resonance cholangiopancreatography in the diagnosis of pancreas divisum: a tertiary center experience. Pancreas 2013;42(3):436–41.
55. Sandrasegaran K, Cote GA, Tahir B, et al. The utility of secretin-enhanced MRCP in diagnosing congenital anomalies. Abdom Imaging 2014;39(5): 979–87.
56. Lans J, Geenen J, Johanson J, et al. Endoscopic therapy in patients with pancreas divisum and acute pancreatitis: a prospective, randomized, controlled clinical trial. Gastrointest Endosc 1992;38(4):430–4.
57. Heyries L, Barthet M, Delvasto C, et al. Long-term results of endoscopic management of pancreas divisum with recurrent acute pancreatitis. Gastrointest Endosc 2002;55(3):376–81.
58. Borak GD, Romagnuolo J, Alsolaiman M, et al. Long-term clinical outcomes after endoscopic minor papilla therapy in symptomatic patients with pancreas divisum. Pancreas 2009;38(8):903–6.
59. Kanth R, Samji NS, Inaganti A, et al. Endotherapy in symptomatic pancreas divisum: A systematic review. Pancreatology 2014;14(4):244–50.
60. Yaghoobi M, Rolland S, Waschke K, et al. Meta-analysis: rectal indomethacin for the prevention of post-ERCP pancreatitis. Aliment Pharmacol Ther 2013;38(9): 995–1001.
61. Petersen BT. An evidence-based review of sphincter of Oddi dysfunction: part I, presentations with "objective" biliary findings (types I and II). Gastrointest Endosc 2004;59(4):525–34.
62. Geenen JE, Hogan WJ, Dodds WJ, et al. The efficacy of endoscopic sphincterotomy after cholecystectomy in patients with sphincter-of-Oddi dysfunction. N Engl J Med 1989;320(2):82–7.
63. Toouli J, Roberts-Thomson IC, Kellow J, et al. Manometry based randomised trial of endoscopic sphincterotomy for sphincter of Oddi dysfunction. Gut 2000;46(1):98–102.

64. Viceconte G, Micheletti A. Endoscopic manometry of the sphincter of Oddi: its usefulness for the diagnosis and treatment of benign papillary stenosis. Scand J Gastroenterol 1995;30(8):797–803.
65. Thatcher BS, Sivak MV, Tedesco FJ, et al. Endoscopic sphincterotomy for suspected dysfunction of the sphincter of Oddi. Gastrointest Endosc 1987; 33(2):91–5.
66. Cicala M, Habib FI, Vavassori P, et al. Outcome of endoscopic sphincterotomy in post cholecystectomy patients with sphincter of Oddi dysfunction as predicted by manometry and quantitative choledochoscintigraphy. Gut 2002;50(5):665–8.
67. Brand B, Wiese L, Thonke F, et al. Outcome of endoscopic sphincterotomy in patients with pain of suspected biliary or papillary origin and inconclusive cholangiography findings. Endoscopy 2001;33(5):405–8.
68. Wilcox CM. Endoscopic therapy for sphincter of Oddi dysfunction in idiopathic pancreatitis: from empiric to scientific. Gastroenterology 2012;143(6):1423–6.
69. Cotton PB, Durkalski V, Romagnuolo J, et al. Effect of endoscopic sphincterotomy for suspected sphincter of Oddi dysfunction on pain-related disability following cholecystectomy: the EPISOD randomized clinical trial. JAMA 2014; 311(20):2101–9.
70. Mosko JD, Chuttani R. EPISOD puts an end to sphincter of Oddi dysfunction type III. Ann Gastroenterol 2014;27(4):427.
71. Coté GA, Imperiale TF, Schmidt SE, et al. Similar efficacies of biliary, with or without pancreatic, sphincterotomy in treatment of idiopathic recurrent acute pancreatitis. Gastroenterology 2012;143(6):1502–9.e1.
72. Hogan WJ, Geenen JE. Biliary dyskinesia. Endoscopy 1988;20(Suppl 1):179–83.
73. Sherman S, Troiano FP, Hawes RH, et al. Frequency of abnormal sphincter of Oddi manometry compared with the clinical suspicion of sphincter of Oddi dysfunction. Am J Gastroenterol 1991;86(5):586–90.
74. Okolo PI, Pasricha PJ, Kalloo AN. What are the long-term results of endoscopic pancreatic sphincterotomy? Gastrointest Endosc 2000;52(1):15–9.
75. Wehrmann T. Long-term results (>/= 10 years) of endoscopic therapy for sphincter of Oddi dysfunction in patients with acute recurrent pancreatitis. Endoscopy 2011;43(3):202–7.
76. Elton E, Howell DA, Parsons WG, et al. Endoscopic pancreatic sphincterotomy: indications, outcome, and a safe stentless technique. Gastrointest Endosc 1998;47(3):240–9.
77. Gupta V, Toskes PP. Diagnosis and management of chronic pancreatitis. Postgrad Med J 2005;81(958):491–7.
78. Axon AT, Classen M, Cotton PB, et al. Pancreatography in chronic pancreatitis: international definitions. Gut 1984;25(10):1107–12.
79. Anand B, Vij J, Mac H, et al. Effect of aging on the pancreatic ducts: a study based on endoscopic retrograde pancreatography. Gastrointest Endosc 1989;35(3):210–3.
80. Hastier P, Buckley MJ, Dumas R, et al. A study of the effect of age on pancreatic duct morphology. Gastrointest Endosc 1998;48(1):53–7.
81. Hastier P, Buckley MJ, Francois E, et al. A prospective study of pancreatic disease in patients with alcoholic cirrhosis: comparative diagnostic value of ERCP and EUS and long-term significance of isolated parenchymal abnormalities. Gastrointest Endosc 1999;49(6):705–9.
82. Dumonceau JM, Delhaye M, Tringali A, et al. Endoscopic treatment of chronic pancreatitis: European Society of Gastrointestinal Endoscopy (ESGE) clinical guideline. Endoscopy 2012;44(8):784–800.

83. Seicean A, Vultur S. Endoscopic therapy in chronic pancreatitis: current perspectives. Clin Exp Gastroenterol 2015;8:1.
84. Cahen DL, Gouma DJ, Nio Y, et al. Endoscopic versus surgical drainage of the pancreatic duct in chronic pancreatitis. N Engl J Med 2007;356(7): 676–84.
85. Maisonneuve P, Lowenfels AB, Mullhaupt B, et al. Cigarette smoking accelerates progression of alcoholic chronic pancreatitis. Gut 2005;54(4):510–4.
86. Rosch T, Daniel S, Scholz M, et al. Endoscopic treatment of chronic pancreatitis: a multicenter study of 1000 patients with long-term follow-up. Endoscopy 2002; 34(10):765–71.
87. Delhaye M, Matos C, Devière J. Endoscopic management of chronic pancreatitis. Gastrointest Endosc Clin N Am 2003;13(4):717–42.
88. Tandan M, Reddy DN. Endotherapy in chronic pancreatitis. World J Gastroenterol 2013;19(37):6156.
89. Costamagna G, Gabbrielli A, Mutignani M, et al. Extracorporeal shock wave lithotripsy of pancreatic stones in chronic pancreatitis: immediate and medium-term results. Gastrointest Endosc 1997;46(3):231–6.
90. Munigala S, Kanwal F, Xian H, et al. New diagnosis of chronic pancreatitis: risk of missing an underlying pancreatic cancer. Am J Gastroenterol 2014;109(11): 1824–30.
91. Nguyen-Tang T, Dumonceau J. Endoscopic treatment in chronic pancreatitis, timing, duration and type of intervention. Best Pract Res Clin Gastroenterol 2010;24(3):281–98.
92. Buscaglia JM, Kalloo AN. Pancreatic sphincterotomy: technique, indications, and complications. World J Gastroenterol 2007;13(30):4064–71.
93. Sherman S, Lehman GA. Endoscopic pancreatic sphincterotomy: techniques and complications. Gastrointest Endosc Clin N Am 1998;8(1):115–24.
94. Sauer BG, Gurka MJ, Ellen K, et al. Effect of pancreatic duct stent diameter on hospitalization in chronic pancreatitis: does size matter? Pancreas 2009;38(7): 728–31.
95. Morgan DE, Smith JK, Hawkins K, et al. Endoscopic stent therapy in advanced chronic pancreatitis: relationships between ductal changes, clinical response, and stent patency. Am J Gastroenterol 2003;98(4):821–6.
96. Costamagna G, Bulajic M, Tringali A, et al. Multiple stenting of refractory pancreatic duct strictures in severe chronic pancreatitis: long-term results. Endoscopy 2006;38(3):254–9.
97. Moon S, Kim M, Park DH, et al. Modified fully covered self-expandable metal stents with antimigration features for benign pancreatic-duct strictures in advanced chronic pancreatitis, with a focus on the safety profile and reducing migration. Gastrointest Endosc 2010;72(1):86–91.
98. Binmoeller KF, Jue P, Seifert H, et al. Endoscopic pancreatic stent drainage in chronic pancreatitis and a dominant stricture: long-term results. Endoscopy 1995;27(9):638–44.
99. Smits ME, Badiga SM, Rauws EA, et al. Long-term results of pancreatic stents in chronic pancreatitis. Gastrointest Endosc 1995;42(5):461–7.
100. Ponchon T, Bory RM, Hedelius F, et al. Endoscopic stenting for pain relief in chronic pancreatitis: results of a standardized protocol. Gastrointest Endosc 1995;42(5):452–6.
101. Seza K, Yamaguchi T, Ishihara T, et al. A long-term controlled trial of endoscopic pancreatic stenting for treatment of main pancreatic duct stricture in chronic pancreatitis. Hepatogastroenterology 2011;58(112):2128–31.

102. Eleftherladis N, Dinu F, Delhaye M, et al. Long-term outcome after pancreatic stenting in severe chronic pancreatitis. Endoscopy 2005;37(3):223–30.
103. Ishihara T, Yamaguchi T, Seza K, et al. Efficacy of s-type stents for the treatment of the main pancreatic duct stricture in patients with chronic pancreatitis. Scand J Gastroenterol 2006;41(6):744–50.
104. Adler DG, Lichtenstein D, Baron TH, et al. The role of endoscopy in patients with chronic pancreatitis. Gastrointest Endosc 2006;63(7):933–7.
105. Johanson JF, Schmalz MJ, Geenen JE. Incidence and risk factors for biliary and pancreatic stent migration. Gastrointest Endosc 1992;38(3):341–6.
106. Ueno N, Hashimoto M, Ozawa Y, et al. Treatment of pancreatic duct stones with the use of endoscopic balloon sphincter dilation. Gastrointest Endosc 1998; 47(3):309–10.
107. Smits ME, Rauws EA, Tytgat GN, et al. Endoscopic treatment of pancreatic stones in patients with chronic pancreatitis. Gastrointest Endosc 1996;43(6): 556–60.
108. Dumonceau J, Devière J, Le Moine O, et al. Endoscopic pancreatic drainage in chronic pancreatitis associated with ductal stones: long-term results. Gastrointest Endosc 1996;43(6):547–55.
109. Lehman GA. Role of ERCP and other endoscopic modalities in chronic pancreatitis. Gastrointest Endosc 2002;56(6):S237–40.
110. Adamek HE, Jakobs R, Buttmann A, et al. Long term follow up of patients with chronic pancreatitis and pancreatic stones treated with extracorporeal shock wave lithotripsy. Gut 1999;45(3):402–5.
111. Dumonceau JM, Costamagna G, Tringali A, et al. Treatment for painful calcified chronic pancreatitis: extracorporeal shock wave lithotripsy versus endoscopic treatment: a randomised controlled trial. Gut 2007;56(4):545–52.
112. Kondo H, Naitoh I, Ohara H, et al. Efficacy of pancreatic stenting prior to extracorporeal shock wave lithotripsy for pancreatic stones. Dig Liver Dis 2014;46(7): 639–44.
113. Tandan M, Reddy DN, Santosh D, et al. Extracorporeal shock wave lithotripsy and endotherapy for pancreatic calculi—a large single center experience. Indian J Gastroenterol 2010;29(4):143–8.
114. Guda NM, Partington S, Freeman ML. Extracorporeal shock wave lithotripsy in the management of chronic calcific pancreatitis: a meta-analysis. JOP 2005; 6(1):6–12.
115. Darisetty S, Tandan M, Reddy DN, et al. Epidural anesthesia is effective for extracorporeal shock wave lithotripsy of pancreatic and biliary calculi. World J Gastrointest Surg 2010;2(5):165–8.
116. Seven G, Schreiner MA, Ross AS, et al. Long-term outcomes associated with pancreatic extracorporeal shock wave lithotripsy for chronic calcific pancreatitis. Gastrointest Endosc 2012;75(5):997–1004.e1.
117. Howell DA, Dy RM, Hanson BL, et al. Endoscopic treatment of pancreatic duct stones using a 10F pancreatoscope and electrohydraulic lithotripsy. Gastrointest Endosc 1999;50(6):829–33.
118. Attwell AR, Brauer BC, Chen YK, et al. Endoscopic retrograde cholangiopancreatography with per oral pancreatoscopy for calcific chronic pancreatitis using endoscope and catheter-based pancreatoscopes: a 10-year single-center experience. Pancreas 2014;43(2):268–74.
119. Attwell AR, Patel S, Kahaleh M, et al. ERCP with per-oral pancreatoscopy-guided laser lithotripsy for calcific chronic pancreatitis: a multicenter US experience. Gastrointest Endosc 2015;82(2):311–8.

120. Parsi MA, Stevens T, Bhatt A, et al. Digital, catheter-based single-operator chol-angiopancreatoscopes: can pancreatoscopy and cholangioscopy become routine procedures? Gastroenterology 2015. [Epub ahead of print].

121. Park DH, Kim MH, Chari ST. Recent advances in autoimmune pancreatitis. Gut 2009;58(12):1680–9.

122. Chari ST, Smyrk TC, Levy MJ, et al. Diagnosis of autoimmune pancreatitis: the Mayo Clinic experience. Clin Gastroenterol Hepatol 2006;4(8):1010–6.

123. Sah RP, Chari ST, Pannala R, et al. Differences in clinical profile and relapse rate of type 1 versus type 2 autoimmune pancreatitis. Gastroenterology 2010;139(1): 140–8.

124. Hamano H, Kawa S, Horiuchi A, et al. High serum IgG4 concentrations in patients with sclerosing pancreatitis. N Engl J Med 2001;344(10):732–8.

125. Kamisawa T, Egawa N, Nakajima H. Autoimmune pancreatitis is a systemic autoimmune disease. Am J Gastroenterol 2003;98(12):2811–2.

126. Maire F, Le Baleur Y, Rebours V, et al. Outcome of patients with type 1 or 2 autoimmune pancreatitis. Am J Gastroenterol 2011;106(1):151–6.

127. Shimosegawa T, Chari ST, Frulloni L, et al. International consensus diagnostic criteria for autoimmune pancreatitis: guidelines of the International Association of Pancreatology. Pancreas 2011;40(3):352–8.

128. Sugumar A, Levy MJ, Kamisawa T, et al. Endoscopic retrograde pancreatogra-phy criteria to diagnose autoimmune pancreatitis: an international multicentre study. Gut 2011;60(5):666–70.

129. Kamisawa T, Tu Y, Egawa N, et al. A new diagnostic endoscopic tool for autoim-mune pancreatitis. Gastrointest Endosc 2008;68(2):358–61.

130. Bhasin DK, Rana SS, Rawal P. Endoscopic retrograde pancreatography in pancreatic trauma: need to break the mental barrier. J Gastroenterol Hepatol 2009;24(5):720–8.

131. Kozarek RA. Endoscopic therapy of complete and partial pancreatic duct disruptions. Gastrointest Endosc Clin N Am 1998;8(1):39–53.

132. Varadarajulu S, Wilcox CM. Endoscopic placement of permanent indwelling transmural stents in disconnected pancreatic duct syndrome: does benefit outweigh the risks? Gastrointest Endosc 2011;74(6):1408–12.

133. Baron TH, Morgan DE. Acute necrotizing pancreatitis. N Engl J Med 1999; 340(18):1412–7.

134. Gillams A, Kurzawinski T, Lees W. Diagnosis of duct disruption and assessment of pancreatic leak with dynamic secretin-stimulated MR cholangiopancreatogra-phy. Am J Roentgenol 2006;186(2):499–506.

135. O'Toole D, Vullierme M, Ponsot P, et al. Diagnosis and management of pancre-atic fistulae resulting in pancreatic ascites or pleural effusions in the era of helical CT and magnetic resonance imaging. Gastroenterol Clin Biol 2007; 31(8):686–93.

136. Bassi C, Dervenis C, Butturini G, et al. Postoperative pancreatic fistula: an inter-national study group (ISGPF) definition. Surgery 2005;138(1):8–13.

137. Brugge WR, Lewandrowski K, Lee-Lewandrowski E, et al. Diagnosis of pancreatic cystic neoplasms: a report of the cooperative pancreatic cyst study. Gastroenter-ology 2004;126(5):1330–6.

138. Kaman L, Behera A, Singh R, et al. Internal pancreatic fistulas with pancreatic ascites and pancreatic pleural effusions: recognition and management. ANZ J Surg 2001;71(4):221–5.

139. Telford JJ, Farrell JJ, Saltzman JR, et al. Pancreatic stent placement for duct disruption. Gastrointest Endosc 2002;56(1):18–24.

140. Varadarajulu S, Noone TC, Tutuian R, et al. Predictors of outcome in pancreatic duct disruption managed by endoscopic transpapillary stent placement. Gastrointest Endosc 2005;61(4):568–75.
141. Lakhtakia S, Reddy DN. Pancreatic leaks: endo-therapy first? J Gastroenterol Hepatol 2009;24(7):1158–60.
142. Catalano MF, Sahai A, Levy M, et al. EUS-based criteria for the diagnosis of chronic pancreatitis: the Rosemont classification. Gastrointest Endosc 2009; 69(7):1251–61.
143. Baron TH, Harewood GC, Morgan DE, et al. Outcome differences after endoscopic drainage of pancreatic necrosis, acute pancreatic pseudocysts, and chronic pancreatic pseudocysts. Gastrointest Endosc 2002;56(1):7–17.
144. Siegel R, Naishadham D, Jemal A. Cancer statistics, 2012. CA Cancer J Clin 2012;62(1):10–29.
145. Kruse EJ. Palliation in pancreatic cancer. Surg Clin North Am 2010;90(2):355–64.
146. Dumonceau JM, Tringali A, Blero D, et al. Biliary stenting: indications, choice of stents and results: European Society of Gastrointestinal Endoscopy (ESGE) clinical guideline. Endoscopy 2012;44(3):277–98.
147. van der Gaag NA, Rauws EA, van Eijck CH, et al. Preoperative biliary drainage for cancer of the head of the pancreas. N Engl J Med 2010;362(2):129–37.
148. Fang Y, Gurusamy KS, Wang Q, et al. Pre-operative biliary drainage for obstructive jaundice. Cochrane Database Syst Rev 2012;9:CD005444.
149. Sugiyama H, Tsuyuguchi T, Sakai Y, et al. Current status of preoperative drainage for distal biliary obstruction. World J Hepatol 2015;7(18):2171.
150. Conroy T, Desseigne F, Ychou M, et al. FOLFIRINOX versus gemcitabine for metastatic pancreatic cancer. N Engl J Med 2011;364(19):1817–25.
151. Boulay BR, Gardner TB, Gordon SR. Occlusion rate and complications of plastic biliary stent placement in patients undergoing neoadjuvant chemoradiotherapy for pancreatic cancer with malignant biliary obstruction. J Clin Gastroenterol 2010;44(6):452–5.
152. Adams MA, Anderson MA, Myles JD, et al. Self-expanding metal stents (SEMS) provide superior outcomes compared to plastic stents for pancreatic cancer patients undergoing neoadjuvant therapy. J Gastrointest Oncol 2012;3(4):309.
153. Moss AC, Morris E, Mac Mathuna P. Palliative biliary stents for obstructing pancreatic carcinoma. Cochrane Database Syst Rev 2006;(2):CD004200.
154. Soderlund C, Linder S. Covered metal versus plastic stents for malignant common bile duct stenosis: a prospective, randomized, controlled trial. Gastrointest Endosc 2006;63(7):986–95.
155. Moss AC, Morris E, Leyden J, et al. Do the benefits of metal stents justify the costs? A systematic review and meta-analysis of trials comparing endoscopic stents for malignant biliary obstruction. Eur J Gastroenterol Hepatol 2007;19(12):1119–24.

Pancreatic Cystic Neoplasms: An Update

Gyanprakash A. Ketwaroo, MD, MSc[a], Koenraad J. Mortele, MD[b],
Mandeep S. Sawhney, MD, MS[c],*

KEYWORDS

- Pancreas • Cystic neoplasm • Mucinous • Cyst

KEY POINTS

- Cystic neoplasms of the pancreas have diverse presentations, varying malignant potential, and with the uncertain natural history of some of these lesions, an evidence-based approach to management is limited.
- There is significant potential for improving the differential diagnosis of cystic neoplasms of the pancreas based on the detection of genetic mutations within cyst fluid.
- There are now several guidelines for the management of cystic neoplasms of the pancreas, each with its own limitations.

INTRODUCTION

Pancreatic cystic neoplasms were historically considered a rare subset of pancreatic tumors. However, the incidence of these lesions is rising, in part from detection through the increasing use of high-resolution cross-sectional imaging techniques.[1] The reported prevalence of pancreatic cystic lesions on imaging studies ranges from 2% to 16%, and increases with advancing age.[2,3] These cystic neoplasms of the pancreas are diverse and can be benign or frankly malignant. Given the rising incidence of cystic pancreatic neoplasms and the demonstrated malignant potential of certain subtypes, accurate diagnosis and multidisciplinary management is paramount.

Initial diagnosis of cystic pancreatic lesions is generally based on imaging characteristics identified on computed tomography (CT) and/or MRI. Endoscopic ultrasound (EUS) provides further imaging characterization, often with increased resolution, and also enables fluid aspiration and analysis to additionally aid differentiation. Cyst fluid

Disclosures: The authors have no conflicts of interest and nothing to disclose.
[a] Division of Gastroenterology, Baylor College of Medicine, Houston, TX, USA; [b] Division of Abdominal Imaging, Department of Radiology, Beth Israel Deaconess Medical Center, Harvard Medical School, Boston, MA, USA; [c] Division of Gastroenterology, Beth Israel Deaconess Medical Center, Harvard Medical School, Boston, MA, USA
* Corresponding author. 330 Brookline Avenue, Rabb-Rose 101, Boston, MA 02215.
E-mail address: msawhney@bidmc.harvard.edu

analysis commonly involves biochemical and cytologic characterization, and in certain cases, assessment for genetic mutations. After diagnosis, the general approach to these lesions includes surgical intervention and/or surveillance imaging. Taking into account diverse presentations, varying malignant potential, and the uncertain natural history of some of these lesions, an evidence-based approach is limited. Consensus guidelines by experts attempt to bridge this gap, and research is ongoing. This article discusses recent updates in the diagnosis and management of cystic neoplasms of the pancreas.

TYPES OF PANCREATIC CYSTIC NEOPLASMS
Serous Cystadenoma

Serous cystadenomas constitute 1% to 2% of exocrine pancreatic tumors with 80% found in women older than 60 years and are therefore sometimes referred to as the "grandmother" tumors.[4] This lesion is considered benign and is typically found incidentally. Occasionally, larger tumors can cause mass effect on surrounding structures, leading to symptoms, such as nausea or abdominal discomfort.[4,5]

Serous cystadenomas are comprised of multiple cysts usually measuring less than 2 cm in size and separated by thin septations that are lined by epithelial cells (Figs. 1–3). The appearance is often described as a "cluster of grapes."[6] On cyst fluid analysis, hemosiderin-laden macrophages are seen histologically in 43% of cases.[7] Characteristically, the cyst fluid has low levels of amylase (<250 IU/L), carcinoembryonic antigen (CEA; <5 ng/mL), and serum carbohydrate-associated antigen 19.9 (CA-19.9; <37 U/mL).[8]

Recent research into serous cystadenomas has focused on their pathogenesis. Clinical case series have suggested an association with von Hippel-Lindau disease, which may implicate a mutation in this gene.[9]

Given the benign nature of the serous cystadenoma, no further follow-up is needed for small cysts once a diagnosis has been made. Larger cysts may demonstrate an increased rate of growth (approximately 2 cm per year), and should be followed

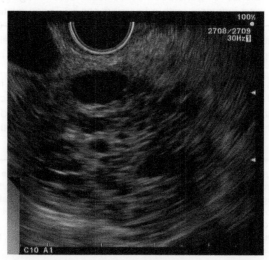

Fig. 1. A 5-cm cyst, composed mostly of microcysts with a honeycombed appearance, is shown on EUS. A few larger 4- to 8-mm cysts are also seen. This appearance is characteristic for a serous cystadenoma.

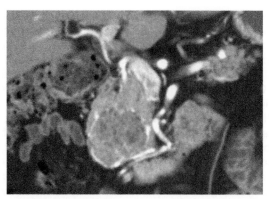

Fig. 2. Coronal contrast-enhanced CT image with a vascular 6-cm lobulated cystic pancreatic lesion in the pancreatic head composed of numerous microcysts. This represented a serous microcystic pancreatic adenoma.

with serial imaging to determine need for resection.[10] The interval and length of time surveillance imaging should be conducted remains unknown.

Intraductal Papillary Mucinous Neoplasm

Intraductal papillary mucinous neoplasms (IPMN) are mucin-producing tumors that were first described as a distinct pancreatic neoplasm in 1982. They may arise from the main duct (main-duct IPMN), the side-branches of the main pancreatic duct (side-branch IPMN), or both (combined-type or mixed IPMN). IPMNs demonstrate a variable natural history, from slow-growing, local lesions to invasive and metastatic tumors. There is geographic variation with regard to distribution of IPMN among the sexes. The mean age of diagnosis is approximately 65 years.

Histologically, an IPMN is characterized by the growth of intraductal mucin-producing columnar cells with differing degrees of dysplasia, and supported by pancreatic parenchyma with fibroatrophic changes. These lesions distend the

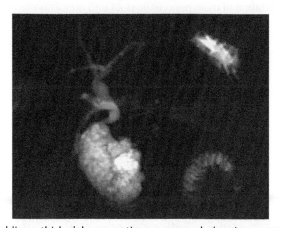

Fig. 3. Coronal oblique thick slab magnetic resonance cholangiopancreatography image shows normal main pancreatic duct and common bile duct but presence of an 8-cm lobulated microcystic mass in the head of the pancreas. This represented a serous microcystic pancreatic adenoma.

affected pancreatic duct with mucin. In the case of side-branch IPMNs, this gives the appearance of a pleomorphic cystic mass in the pancreas that communicates with the main pancreatic duct (**Fig. 4**). Identifying this communication is important, because other neoplastic cystic neoplasms generally do not communicate with the pancreatic duct. Main-duct IPMNs are characterized by a focal or diffuse dilation of the main pancreatic duct. Combined duct IPMNs have features of both main-duct and side-branch IPMNs (**Fig. 5**).

Side-branch IPMNs are commonly found in the uncinate process, but can be seen throughout the pancreas. They may be solitary or multiple. Given the importance of demonstrating connection of the cyst to the main pancreatic duct, magnetic resonance cholangiopancreatography (MRCP) and EUS have emerged as important noninvasive ways of making the diagnosis. Arakawa and colleagues[11] have also demonstrated that findings made on MRCP may correlate with findings at histopathology.

IPMN cyst fluid may stain positive for alcian blue and mucicarmine, highlighting the presence of mucin. IPMNs may have a variable amylase level, reflecting communication with the pancreatic duct, and a high CEA level (>200 ng/mL).[12]

IPMNs are further classified into intestinal, pancreaticobiliary, gastric, and oncocytic-types. This classification is highly predictive of their biologic behavior, but of limited clinical use because preoperative determination of subtype is presently not possible.[13] The main-duct IPMN is primarily of the intestinal-type and is considered highly likely to harbor malignancy. Resection is thus recommended for all patients with main-duct IPMN. However, recent studies have suggested that there may be substantial variation in malignant potential of main-duct IPMNs. In a small study by Abdeljawad and colleagues,[14] absence of symptoms and main duct size less than 8 mm was associated with a lower malignancy risk (25% vs 69%).

The side-branch IPMN is considered less likely to harbor or develop into malignancy and management often includes surveillance after risk stratification (discussed in detail later). Mixed-type IPMN have features of both side-branch and main-duct IPMN. These are thought to have the same malignant potential as main-duct IPMN. A study by Sahora and colleagues[15] suggested that a subset of mixed-type IPMN, which they termed minimal mixed-type IPMN (defined as absence of gross abnormalities except for dilatation of main pancreatic duct and noncircumferential microscopic

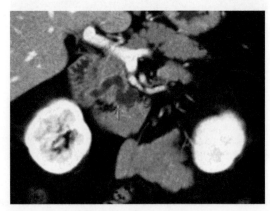

Fig. 4. Coronal contrast-enhanced CT image shows a 2-cm cystic pancreatic lesion (*arrows*) in the uncinate process connecting with the main pancreatic duct that is dilated up to the papilla. This represented a side-branch IPMN.

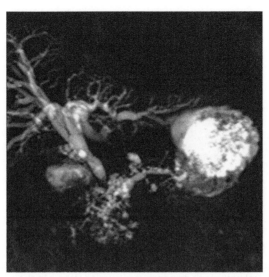

Fig. 5. Coronal oblique thick slab magnetic resonance cholangiopancreatography image shows dilated and obstructed common bile duct and dilated main pancreatic duct with multiple associated side-branch lesions. This represented malignant combined duct IPMN.

involvement of main pancreatic duct), may be biologically similar to side-branch IPMN both with regard to demonstrating gastric-type epithelium and low risk of malignant transformation.

There is ongoing research into additional noninvasive markers of high-risk IPMNs. Recently, researchers have identified serum N-glycan as a potential biomarker. In a study of 79 patients with IPMNs, 13 of which were invasive, high levels of fucosylated complex-type glycans, especially m/z 3195, correlated with invasive IPMN.[16] Yabusaki and colleagues[17] have also identified a polymorphism in the vascular endothelial growth factor gene (VEGF) as associated with malignant transformation in IPMNs. Analysis of the secretin-stimulated pancreatic juice collected from the duodenum may also provide insight into patients with IPMNs who have high-grade dysplasia or even pancreatic cancer. Studies, albeit in heterogeneous populations, have identified TP53, GNAS, and KRAS in pancreatic juice as potential candidate genes.[18–20]

Mucinous Cystic Neoplasm

Mucinous cystic neoplasms (MCN) account for approximately 2.5% of exocrine pancreatic tumors. These occur almost exclusively in women (99.7%) with a mean age of occurrence of 50 (range, 20–82 years).[21–23] Therefore, these have often been referred to as the "mother" cyst. They are commonly found in the pancreatic body and tail, because of the close proximity of the female gonad to the pancreatic tail during embryologic life. MCN include the benign but potentially premalignant mucinous cystadenoma; borderline MCN; MCN with carcinoma in situ; and the most aggressive form, mucinous cystadenocarcinoma.[22,23]

MCN are characterized by an encapsulated and dominant round or oval cyst, with average sizes ranging from 6 cm to 11 cm.[24] Histologically, the cyst is comprised of ovarian-type stroma, unique among the cystic neoplasms, with epithelial elements consisting of tall columnar cells with abundant intracellular mucin (**Fig. 6**).

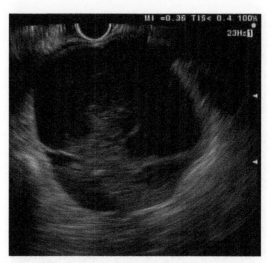

Fig. 6. A 5-cm cystic mass with well-defined borders is shown on EUS. A solid mass is noted within the cyst. Surgical pathology demonstrated ovarian stroma in the cyst wall, confirming the diagnosis of mucinous cystic neoplasm. The solid mass within the cyst was an adenocarcinoma.

On CT and MRI studies, enhancement of the capsule along with enhancement of any septations or mural nodules is depicted after administration of contrast material (**Figs. 7** and **8**).[25] As with IPMN, cyst fluid may stain positive for alcian blue and muci-carmine, highlighting the presence of mucin. On cyst fluid analysis, there is a variable amylase level, typically a high CEA (>800 ng/mL) level and, when malignant, also an elevated CA-19.9 level.[26]

With MCN, there is significant histopathologic variation, with portions of relatively benign-appearing epithelium adjacent to areas of invasive carcinoma. Thus, a biopsy to determine benign versus invasive disease is unreliable. Given the malignant potential of these lesions, and the relatively young age at diagnosis, surgery is traditionally

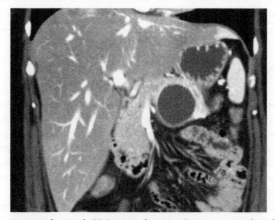

Fig. 7. Coronal contrast-enhanced CT image shows a 5-cm encapsulated cystic pancreatic lesion in the pancreatic body without associated main duct dilation. This represented a benign MCN.

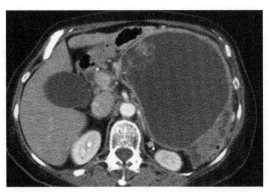

Fig. 8. Axial contrast-enhanced CT image shows a 5-cm encapsulated cystic pancreatic lesion in the pancreatic tail with soft tissue component. This represented a dysplastic MCN.

considered for all patients. Although imaging characteristics (solitary, location, presence of capsule, and no communication with the main pancreatic duct) often distinguish a MCN from an IPMN, a study by Nagashio and colleagues[27] suggested that a combination of cyst fluid CEA and CA-125 may also aid in distinguishing these two entities.

Solid Pseudopapillary Neoplasm

The solid pseudopapillary neoplasm (SPN), formerly known as solid and papillary epithelial neoplasm, is a rare pancreatic tumor with less than 1000 cases described in the literature. SPN occurs most commonly in young (mean age, 25 years) women (85%). Recent data have highlighted specific molecular aberrations in the pathogenesis of SPN including CTNNB1 mutations and activation of the Wnt/beta-catenin pathway, distinct from the KRAS, TP53, and SMAD4 mutations typically observed in pancreatic ductal adenocarcinoma.[28]

SPNs are generally benign or low-grade malignant tumors. As with serous cystadenomas, large SPNs can become symptomatic because of mass effect on surrounding structures. On CT, SPNs are generally characterized as well-demarcated, encapsulated, large, cystic and solid masses. In cystic and solid tumors, the solid tissue components are generally noted at the periphery, with central areas of hemorrhage and cystic degeneration noted more centrally. A key diagnostic finding of SPN is the presence of a fibrous capsule that encompasses and surrounds the tumor. Postcontrast administration, the capsule and solid components enhance on CT and MRI. EUS/fine-needle aspiration (FNA) is important in the diagnosis of this lesion, increasing the diagnostic yield to more than 80% and also assisting in risk stratification. In a small retrospective study, focal discontinuity of the capsule on imaging was associated with malignancy.[29] In a retrospective study of 97 patients who underwent resection, positive reactivity to Ki-67 was more common in tumors with malignancy.[30]

SPNs, because of their large size at presentation and possible malignant potential, are generally resected. Occasionally, enucleation has been performed, made possible by the fibrous capsule encompassing the tumor.[31] Overall, patients with this tumor have excellent prognoses with a 5-year survival of 95%.[32] More minimally invasive surgical resection also seems to have similarly excellent outcomes.[33] However, recurrence can occur in almost 10% of patients after 5 years, and thus long-term follow-up is essential. Lymphovascular invasion, synchronous metastases, and local invasion of the tumor capsule are associated with late recurrence.[34]

DISTINGUISHING BETWEEN CYSTIC NEOPLASMS

Patient demographics, location and number of cysts, presence or absence of a capsule, and cyst fluid analysis are useful features that help distinguish between cysts and are detailed in **Table 1**. In a recent multicenter, retrospective study of 130 patients with resected pancreatic cystic neoplasms, primarily IPMNs but also including serous cystadenomas, solid-pseudopapillary neoplasms, and MCN, cyst fluid was analyzed to identify subtle genetic mutations.[35] An algorithm based on mutations and other aberrations in these genes (BRAF, CDKN2A, CTNNB1, GNAS, KRAS, NRAS, PIK3CA, RNF43, SMAD4, TP53, and VHL) and clinical features was able to classify cyst type with 90% to 100% sensitivity and 92% to 98% specificity. This is an important development in the ongoing research into classifying and risk-stratifying cystic pancreatic neoplasms.

MANAGEMENT OF PANCREATIC CYSTS: REVIEW OF CURRENT GUIDELINES

Guidelines for the management of pancreatic cysts have been issued by several different societies, including the American College of Radiology (ACR), the American Gastroenterology Association (AGA), and a group of international experts in pancreatology (known as the Fukuoka guidelines). These guidelines share an emphasis on established risk factors for aggressive behavior of these cysts in guiding surveillance and management strategies. These risk factors include size, especially greater than 3 cm; dilation of the main pancreatic duct; and the presence of a solid component within the cyst or enhancing nodule in the wall of the cyst. The presence of symptoms, such as pancreatitis or obstructive jaundice, also raises the concern for malignancy.

Management of Cysts Less Than 3 cm

The ACR Incidental Findings Committee notes that incidentally found cysts in asymptomatic patients that are less than 2 cm in size have very low incidence of cancer and, therefore, the ACR does not recommend that these lesions be immediately characterized by more detailed imaging.[36] They recommend one follow-up examination, preferable with a limited T2-weighted MRI at a 1-year interval. If the cyst is unchanged, no further follow-up is recommended. For cysts 2 to 3 cm in size, they recommend pancreas-dedicated MRI with MRCP to further characterize the lesion. Based on MRI characteristics, recommendations are as follows: uncharacterized cysts, yearly follow-up; branch-duct IPMN, follow-up every 6 months for 2 years and then yearly; serous cystadenoma, follow-up every 2 years. There are no recommendations on when surveillance can be stopped.

The AGA recommends that patients with pancreatic cysts less than 3 cm without either a solid component or a dilated pancreatic duct undergo MRI for surveillance in 1 year and then every 2 years for a total of 5 years.[37,38] If there is no change in the cyst, then surveillance is stopped at 5 years. The recommendations regarding follow-up intervals are not based on any specific evidence, but are believed to be reasonable given the small absolute risk of malignancy. Using Surveillance, Epidemiology, and End Results database statistics, the authors estimated that a cyst seen incidentally on MRI had only a 1 in 10,000 chance of being a mucinous invasive malignancy, and a 1.7 in 10,000 chance of being a ductal cancer.

International consensus guidelines for the management of IPMN and MCN of the pancreas were updated in 2012, and are commonly referred to as the "Fukuoka" guidelines.[39] These recommend that an attempt be made to differentiate branch-duct IPMN, MCN, and other cysts based on imaging characteristics. For branch-duct IPMNs less than 3 cm that do not exhibit "high-risk stigmata of malignancy" or

Table 1
A comparison of the characteristics of side-branch IPMNs, MCNs, and serous cystadenomas

	Side-branch IPMN	MCN	Serous Cystadenoma
Average age (y)	65	50	60
Gender	Male	Female	Female
Common location in pancreas	Uncinate	Body/tail	Slight predominance in head, but occurs throughout pancreas
Multifocal	Yes	No	No
EUS findings	Communication with main pancreatic duct; Positive "string sign"[a]	Large cyst, with septations, not communicating with main pancreatic duct; May have peripheral calcifications; Positive "string sign"[a]	Honeycomb appearance with multiple septae; Fluid is thin and not viscous
Encapsulated	No	Yes	No
CT/MRI findings	Pleomorphic, communicates with pancreatic duct, pseudoseptations	Round or oval, well-circumscribed with enhancement of capsule; Macrocystic	Lobulated, well circumscribed; Central stellate scar and calcifications; Microcystic
Histology	Mucin-producing columnar cells	Ovarian-like stroma; Tall columnar cells with abundant intracellular mucin	Multiple cysts with thin septae lined with epithelial cells
Cyst fluid CEA level	>200 ng/mL	>800 ng/mL	<5 ng/mL
Amylase	Variable	Variable	<250 IU/L
KRAS mutation	Yes	Yes	No
GNAS mutation	Yes	No	No
Cytology	Viscous, mucin-rich fluid	Viscous, mucin-rich fluid with columnar epithelial cells	Serous fluid with glycogen-staining cuboidal cells

[a] String sign: aspirated cyst fluid viscous and can be pulled into a string.

"worrisome features," recommendations are as follows: cyst size less than 1 cm, CT/MRI in 2 to 3 years; 1 to 2 cm, CT/MRI yearly for 2 years, and then lengthen interval; 2 to 3 cm, EUS in 3 to 6 months, and then lengthen interval alternating MRI with EUS (**Table 2**). These recommendations are the most intensive when compared with other guidelines, and are based on studies from Japan that suggest an increased incidence of pancreatic ductal adenocarcinoma in patients with side-branch IPMN.

The authors of this article do not endorse such intensive follow-up, because it is unclear whether imaging surveillance can detect early ductal adenocarcinoma. Furthermore, the optimal surveillance interval and cost-effectiveness of such an approach is unknown. The guidelines also recommend resection for all MCNs in surgically fit patients. This is based on the rationale that the natural history of MCN is still unknown, and nonoperative management requires years of follow-up resulting in high costs.

Management of Cysts Greater Than 3 cm

The ACR guidelines recommend aspiration and consideration for surgery for cysts greater than 3 cm. Exceptions are made for serous cystadenoma, where surgery is deferred until the cyst is greater than 4 cm; and for solid pseudopapillary epithelial neoplasm, where surgery is recommended for all lesions. The authors of this article do not endorse surgery for all cysts greater than 3 cm.

The AGA guidelines recommend MRI in a year and then every 2 years for asymptomatic cysts that are greater than 3 cm and are not associated with either main pancreatic duct dilation or solid component. For cysts greater than 3 cm, and with

Table 2
Fukuoka guidelines: management of pancreatic cysts based on presence of risk factors

Risk Factors	Management
Presence of high-risk stigmata[a]	Surgical removal of cyst
Presence of worrisome features[b]	Perform endoscopic ultrasound
Worrisome features confirmed on EUS[c]	Surgical removal of cyst
EUS inconclusive for concerning features	Close surveillance alternating EUS with MRI every 3–6 mo Strongly consider surgery in young, fit individuals
Cyst <1 cm and no high-risk stigmata or concerning features on EUS	CT/MRI every 2–3 y
Cyst 1–2 cm and no high-risk stigmata or concerning features on EUS	CT/MRI yearly × 2 y and then lengthen interval if no change
Cyst 2–3 cm and no high-risk stigmata or concerning features on EUS	EUS in 3–6 mo then lengthen interval, alternating with MRI as appropriate Consider surgery in young, fit individuals with need for prolonged surveillance
Cyst >3 cm and no high-risk stigmata or concerning features on EUS	Close surveillance alternating EUS with MRI every 3–6 mo Strongly consider surgery in young, fit individuals

[a] High-risk stigmata: obstructive jaundice with head of pancreas cyst, main pancreatic duct at least 1 cm in size, enhancing solid component within cyst.
[b] Worrisome imaging features: thickened/enhanced cyst walls, cyst at least 3 cm in size, main pancreatic duct 5–9 mm in size, nonenhancing mural nodule, abrupt change in caliber of pancreatic duct with distal pancreatic atrophy. Worrisome clinical features: pancreatitis.
[c] EUS confirmation of worrisome features: definite mural nodule, main pancreatic duct showing features of involvement, cytology suspicious or positive for malignancy.

either main pancreas duct dilation or the presence of solid component, an evaluation with EUS and EUS-guided FNA is recommended. Further management decisions are based on EUS findings and are discussed later.

The Fukuoka guidelines recommend EUS and EUS-guided FNA for all cysts greater than 3 cm. Further decisions are based on EUS findings and are discussed next.

Indication for Surgery

The Fukuoka guidelines recommend surgery for all cysts with "high-risk stigmata of malignancy" (see **Table 2**). These include either obstructive jaundice in patients with cysts in the head of the pancreas, enhancing solid component within cyst, or main pancreatic duct greater than 10 mm in diameter.

The Fukuoka guidelines categorize the following as "worrisome features": cyst greater than 3 cm, thickened/enhancing cyst walls, main pancreatic duct diameter 5 to 9 mm, nonenhancing mural nodule, and abrupt change in caliber of pancreatic duct with distal pancreatic atrophy. These patients should undergo EUS, and surgery should be considered if any of the following features are confirmed on EUS: definite mural nodule, main pancreatic duct features suspicious for involvement, or cytology suspicious or positive for malignancy. Endosonographers must not mistake mucin globules or debris within the cyst for intramural nodules. Features of true tumor nodule include lack of mobility, presence of Doppler flow, and FNA of nodule showing tumor tissue. EUS features suggestive of main pancreas duct involvement are thickened duct walls, intraductal mucin, or mural nodules within the main duct. In the absence of these features, main duct involvement is inconclusive and ongoing surveillance is warranted.

AGA guidelines identified three features that are associated with increased risk for malignancy in pancreatic cysts: (1) cyst size greater than 3 cm (odds ratio [OR], 2.97; 95% confidence interval [CI], 1.82–4.85), (2) presence of a solid component (OR, 7.73; 95% CI, 3.38–17.67), and (3) dilated pancreatic duct (OR, 2.38; 95% CI, 0.71–8.00). Interestingly, increase in the cyst size was not found to predict malignancy. Guidelines recommend consideration for surgery if at least two of three features are confirmed on EUS, or if malignant cyst fluid cytology is found. The AGA does not endorse surgery for all patients with MCN, but does not provide specific guidelines as to when surgery should be considered.

The decision to consider surgery for pancreas cysts is a difficult balancing act and needs to take into account the patient's age, comorbid illnesses, ability for close and reliable follow-up, and local surgical expertise. Sahora and colleagues[40] recently demonstrated that the Charlson Comorbidity Index of greater than 7 correlated with a median survival of 43 months in patients with IPMNs. These patients may thus not be best served by surgery or even IPMN surveillance.

Several important factors were reported by the AGA technical review that should also be kept in mind when counseling patients in this regard. The overall mortality rate for pancreas surgery when done at an expert center was 2.1% (95% CI, 1.5%–2.7%), and was several fold higher (approximately 7%) when outcomes from all centers were assessed. The morbidity rate following pancreas surgery was 30% (95% CI, 25%–35%). Fifty-eight percent (95% CI, 55%–61%) of patients who underwent surgery for pancreatic cysts were found to have only low-risk lesions. However, invasive malignancy was noted in 25% (95% CI, 23%–27%) of surgery patients. The 5-year survival in those without invasive malignancy was 80% to 100%. The 5-year survival dropped to an average of 28% once invasive malignancy developed. The proportion of cases developing invasive malignancy was estimated at 0.72% per year (95% CI, 0.48–1.08). Taken together, these findings suggest that patient selection for surgery remains problematic, with some patients being sent to surgery prematurely, whereas in others surgery is being delayed.

Recent studies have evaluated and compared the 2006 Sendai and the updated 2012 Fukuoka guidelines. A review of 114 surgically treated patients highlighted the superiority of the Fukuoka guidelines in predicting high-grade dysplasia/invasive carcinoma.[41] However, a retrospective review of 194 patients with cystic lesions of the pancreas found no statistical difference in the guidelines for predicting patients with advanced neoplasia.[42] A systematic review of 1382 surgically resected patients by Goh and colleagues[43] showed that some malignant and even invasive IPMNs may be missed with the Fukuoka guidelines. Thus overall, the Fukuoka guidelines seem to add some benefit but may still miss concerning lesions. The AGA guidelines are different from all other guidelines in that they make recommendations on when surveillance can be stopped. These guidelines have presently not been subjected to external validation. Shimizu and colleagues[44] have developed and validated a nomogram for predicting the probability of carcinoma in patients with IPMN. However, its accuracy also needs to be validated in larger cohorts.

Principles of Surgical Resection

The Fukuoka guidelines recommend anatomic pancreas resection with lymph node dissection as the standard surgical approach for mucinous cysts. More limited surgery, such as excision or enucleation, may be considered for mucinous cysts without clinical or radiologic suspicion of malignancy. When available, a minimally invasive approach, such as laparoscopic or robotic surgery, may be appropriate for cysts with low-grade and possibly high-grade dysplasia. Conversion to a standard resection should be considered if operative findings or frozen-section pathology reveals invasive disease. When the final pathology reveals invasion or high-grade dysplasia at the resection margin, a reoperation should be considered.

Follow-Up After Surgery

The AGA guidelines recommend that patients should undergo annual surveillance with MRI after surgical resection of cyst with dysplasia or malignancy. The surveillance should be continued as long as the patient is a surgical candidate. This recommendation is based on the possibility that such patients may be at high risk of developing malignancy because of a field defect involving the entire pancreas; ongoing exposure to risk factors, such as smoking; and genetic predisposition. The AGA does not recommend postoperative surveillance for nondysplastic cysts.

The Fukuoka guidelines recommend repeat examinations at 2 and 5 years to check for new lesions in patients with nondysplastic cysts and negative surgical margins. For patients with noninvasive IPMN and low-grade or moderate-grade dysplasia at the margin, MRCP surveillance twice a year is recommended. Patients with multifocal side-branch IPMNs in whom cysts remain in the pancreas remnant should follow recommendations for nonresected IPMNs.

Extrapancreatic Neoplasms in Patients with Intraductal Papillary Mucinous Neoplasms

Early retrospective studies had suggested an increased incidence of extrapancreatic neoplasms in patients with IPMNs.[45] Subsequent prospective studies including a very recent large multicenter study of 816 patients with IPMNs, followed over 14 years, suggested this was not the case.[46,47] A systematic review by Pugliese and coworkers[48] in 2015 also suggested that the data are lacking for increased extrapancreatic neoplasms in IPMN. Currently, additional surveillance for extrapancreatic malignancy in patients is not recommended.

SUMMARY

Cystic neoplasms of the pancreas comprise an important subset of pancreatic lesions. The varying malignant potential of serous cystadenomas, IPMNs, MCNs, and SPN warrant accurate, minimally invasive diagnosis and multidisciplinary management. Recent research into this field has focused on such an approach to these lesions, leading to the updates described in this article. However, much more work is needed as clinicians move away from consensus documents toward evidence-based diagnosis and management.

REFERENCES

1. Khalid A, Brugge W. ACG practice guidelines for the diagnosis and management of neoplastic pancreatic cysts. Am J Gastroenterol 2007;102(10):2339–49.
2. de Jong K, Bruno MJ, Fockens P. Epidemiology, diagnosis, and management of cystic lesions of the pancreas. Gastroenterol Res Pract 2012;2012:147465.
3. de Jong K, Nio CY, Hermans JJ, et al. High prevalence of pancreatic cysts detected by screening magnetic resonance imaging examinations. Clin Gastroenterol Hepatol 2010;8(9):806–11.
4. Buck JL, Hayes WS. From the archives of the AFIP. Microcystic adenoma of the pancreas. Radiographics 1990;10(2):313–22.
5. Colonna J, Plaza JA, Frankel WL, et al. Serous cystadenoma of the pancreas: clinical and pathological features in 33 patients. Pancreatology 2008;8(2):135–41.
6. Khurana B, Mortelé KJ, Glickman J, et al. Macrocystic serous adenoma of the pancreas: radiologic-pathologic correlation. AJR Am J Roentgenol 2003;181(1): 119–23.
7. Belsley NA, Pitman MB, Lauwers GY, et al. Serous cystadenoma of the pancreas: limitations and pitfalls of endoscopic ultrasound-guided fine-needle aspiration biopsy. Cancer 2008;114(2):102–10.
8. van der Waaij LA, van Dullemen HM, Porte RJ. Cyst fluid analysis in the differential diagnosis of pancreatic cystic lesions: a pooled analysis. Gastrointest Endosc 2005;62(3):383–9.
9. de Mestier L, Hammel P. Pancreatic neuroendocrine tumors in von Hippel-Lindau disease. Scand J Gastroenterol 2015;50(8):1054–5.
10. El-Hayek KM, Brown N, O'Rourke C, et al. Rate of growth of pancreatic serous cystadenoma as an indication for resection. Surgery 2013;154(4):794–800 [discussion: 800–2].
11. Arakawa A, Yamashita Y, Namimoto T, et al. Intraductal papillary tumors of the pancreas. Histopathologic correlation of MR cholangiopancreatography findings. Acta Radiol 2000;41(4):343–7.
12. Park WG, Mascarenhas R, Palaez-Luna M, et al. Diagnostic performance of cyst fluid carcinoembryonic antigen and amylase in histologically confirmed pancreatic cysts. Pancreas 2011;40(1):42–5.
13. Distler M, Kersting S, Niedergethmann M, et al. Pathohistological subtype predicts survival in patients with intraductal papillary mucinous neoplasm (IPMN) of the pancreas. Ann Surg 2013;258(2):324–30.
14. Abdeljawad K, Vemulapalli KC, Schmidt CM, et al. Prevalence of malignancy in patients with pure main duct intraductal papillary mucinous neoplasms. Gastrointest Endosc 2014;79(4):623–9.
15. Sahora K, Fernández-del Castillo C, Dong F, et al. Not all mixed-type intraductal papillary mucinous neoplasms behave like main-duct lesions: implications of minimal involvement of the main pancreatic duct. Surgery 2014;156(3):611–21.

16. Akimoto Y, Nouso K, Kato H, et al. Serum N-glycan profiles in patients with intraductal papillary mucinous neoplasms of the pancreas. Pancreatology 2015;15(4):432–8.
17. Yabusaki N, Yamada S, Shimoyama Y, et al. A vascular endothelial growth factor gene polymorphism predicts malignant potential in intraductal papillary mucinous neoplasm. Pancreas 2015;44(4):608–14.
18. Kanda M, Knight S, Topazian M, et al. Mutant GNAS detected in duodenal collections of secretin-stimulated pancreatic juice indicates the presence or emergence of pancreatic cysts. Gut 2013;62(7):1024–33.
19. Kanda M, Sadakari Y, Borges M, et al. Mutant TP53 in duodenal samples of pancreatic juice from patients with pancreatic cancer or high-grade dysplasia. Clin Gastroenterol Hepatol 2013;11(6):719–30.e5.
20. Eshleman JR, Norris AL, Sadakari Y, et al. KRAS and guanine nucleotide-binding protein mutations in pancreatic juice collected from the duodenum of patients at high risk for neoplasia undergoing endoscopic ultrasound. Clin Gastroenterol Hepatol 2015;13(5):963–9.e4.
21. Scott J, Martin I, Redhead D, et al. Mucinous cystic neoplasms of the pancreas: imaging features and diagnostic difficulties. Clin Radiol 2000;55(3):187–92.
22. Crippa S, Salvia R, Warshaw AL, et al. Mucinous cystic neoplasm of the pancreas is not an aggressive entity: lessons from 163 resected patients. Ann Surg 2008;247(4):571–9.
23. Goh BK, Tan YM, Chung YF, et al. A review of mucinous cystic neoplasms of the pancreas defined by ovarian-type stroma: clinicopathological features of 344 patients. World J Surg 2006;30(12):2236–45.
24. Buetow PC, Rao P, Thompson LD. From the archives of the AFIP. Mucinous cystic neoplasms of the pancreas: radiologic-pathologic correlation. Radiographics 1998;18(2):433–49.
25. Zhong N, Zhang L, Takahashi N, et al. Histologic and imaging features of mural nodules in mucinous pancreatic cysts. Clin Gastroenterol Hepatol 2012;10(2):192–8, 198.e1–2.
26. Bhutani MS, Gupta V, Guha S, et al. Pancreatic cyst fluid analysis: a review. J Gastrointestin Liver Dis 2011;20(2):175–80.
27. Nagashio Y, Hijioka S, Mizuno N, et al. Combination of cyst fluid CEA and CA 125 is an accurate diagnostic tool for differentiating mucinous cystic neoplasms from intraductal papillary mucinous neoplasms. Pancreatology 2014;14(6):503–9.
28. Bhatnagar R, Olson MT, Fishman EK, et al. Solid-pseudopapillary neoplasm of the pancreas: cytomorphologic findings and literature review. Acta Cytol 2014;58(4):347–55.
29. Huang YS, Chen JL, Chang CC, et al. Solid pseudopapillary neoplasms of the pancreas: imaging differentiation between benignity and malignancy. Hepatogastroenterology 2014;61(131):809–13.
30. Yu P, Cheng X, Du Y, et al. Solid pseudopapillary neoplasms of the pancreas: a 19-year multicenter experience in China. J Gastrointest Surg 2015;19(8):1433–40.
31. Karakas S, Dirican A, Soyer V, et al. A pancreatic pseudopapillary tumor enucleated curatively. Int J Surg Case Rep 2015;10:118–20.
32. Li G, Baek NH, Yoo K, et al. Surgical outcomes for solid pseudopapillary neoplasm of the pancreas. Hepatogastroenterology 2014;61(134):1780–4.
33. Graziosi L, Marino E, Rivellini R, et al. Retrospective analysis of short term outcomes after spleen-preserving distal pancreatectomy for solid pseudopapillary tumours. Int J Surg 2015;21(Suppl 1):S26–9.

34. Serrano PE, Serra S, Al-Ali H, et al. Risk factors associated with recurrence in patients with solid pseudopapillary tumors of the pancreas. JOP 2014;15(6):561–8.
35. Springer S, Wang Y, Molin MD, et al. A combination of molecular markers and clinical features improve the classification of pancreatic cysts. Gastroenterology 2015;149(6):1501–10.
36. Berland LL, Silverman SG, Gore RM, et al. Managing incidental findings on abdominal CT: white paper of the ACR incidental findings committee. J Am Coll Radiol 2010;7(10):754–73.
37. Scheiman JM, Hwang JH, Moayyedi P. American Gastroenterological Association technical review on the diagnosis and management of asymptomatic neoplastic pancreatic cysts. Gastroenterology 2015;148(4):824–48.e22.
38. Vege SS, Ziring B, Jain R, et al. American Gastroenterological Association institute guideline on the diagnosis and management of asymptomatic neoplastic pancreatic cysts. Gastroenterology 2015;148(4):819–22 [quiz: e12–3].
39. Tanaka M, Fernández-del Castillo C, Adsay V, et al. International consensus guidelines 2012 for the management of IPMN and MCN of the pancreas. Pancreatology 2012;12(3):183–97.
40. Sahora K, Ferrone CR, Brugge WR, et al. Effects of comorbidities on outcomes of patients with intraductal papillary mucinous neoplasms. Clin Gastroenterol Hepatol 2015;13(10):1816–23.
41. Goh BK, Thng CH, Tan DM, et al. Evaluation of the Sendai and 2012 International Consensus Guidelines based on cross-sectional imaging findings performed for the initial triage of mucinous cystic lesions of the pancreas: a single institution experience with 114 surgically treated patients. Am J Surg 2014;208(2):202–9.
42. Kaimakliotis P, Riff B, Pourmand K, et al. Sendai and Fukuoka consensus guidelines identify advanced neoplasia in patients with suspected mucinous cystic neoplasms of the pancreas. Clin Gastroenterol Hepatol 2015;13(10):1808–15.
43. Goh BK, Lin Z, Tan DM, et al. Evaluation of the Fukuoka consensus guidelines for intraductal papillary mucinous neoplasms of the pancreas: results from a systematic review of 1,382 surgically resected patients. Surgery 2015;158(5):1192–202.
44. Shimizu Y, Yamaue H, Maguchi H, et al. Validation of a nomogram for predicting the probability of carcinoma in patients with intraductal papillary mucinous neoplasm in 180 pancreatic resection patients at 3 high-volume centers. Pancreas 2015;44(3):459–64.
45. Yoon WJ, Ryu JK, Lee JK, et al. Extrapancreatic malignancies in patients with intraductal papillary mucinous neoplasm of the pancreas: prevalence, associated factors, and comparison with patients with other pancreatic cystic neoplasms. Ann Surg Oncol 2008;15(11):3193–8.
46. Kawakubo K, Tada M, Isayama H, et al. Incidence of extrapancreatic malignancies in patients with intraductal papillary mucinous neoplasms of the pancreas. Gut 2011;60(9):1249–53.
47. Marchegiani G, Malleo G, D'Haese JG, et al. Association between pancreatic intraductal papillary mucinous neoplasms and extrapancreatic malignancies. Clin Gastroenterol Hepatol 2015;13(6):1162–9.
48. Pugliese L, Keskin M, Maisonneuve P, et al. Increased incidence of extrapancreatic neoplasms in patients with IPMN: fact or fiction? A critical systematic review. Pancreatology 2015;15(3):209–16.

Islet Cell Tumors of the Pancreas

Sunil Amin, MD, MPH, Michelle Kang Kim, MD, PhD*

KEYWORDS

- Islet cell tumor • Pancreatic neuroendocrine tumors (PNET) • Pancreas
- Pancreas cancer • Targeted molecular therapy

KEY POINTS

- Islet cell tumors of the pancreas, also known as pancreatic neuroendocrine tumors (PNETs), are rare neoplasms that constitute fewer than 5% of pancreatic tumors.
- Although PNETs may present with distinct clinical syndromes, most of these tumors are nonfunctional.
- In a minority of cases, PNETs arise in the background of known genetic syndromes such as multiple endocrine neoplasia type I or von Hippel-Lindau syndrome.
- Surgery remains the cornerstone of treatment, provided that 90% of the tumor burden can be resected.
- For nonresectable well-differentiated lesions, somatostatin analogues, chemotherapy, targeted molecular therapy, and peptide receptor radiotherapy are appropriate options that lead to increased survival.

INTRODUCTION

Islet cell tumors of the pancreas, also known as pancreatic neuroendocrine tumors (PNETs), are a group of tumors that arise from the endocrine pancreas. Although PNETs may produce distinct clinical syndromes, most of these neoplasms are asymptomatic and present as an incidental finding. PNETs are a distinct group of neuroendocrine tumor (NET), with important biological differences from luminal (carcinoid) neoplasms. This article summarizes the important characteristics of PNETs with regard to epidemiology, pathology, diagnosis, and treatment, with a focus on new developments and their potential roles in the evolving management of this disease.

EPIDEMIOLOGY

PNETs are rare neoplasms that constitute fewer than 5% of pancreatic tumors, and only 7% of all NETs.[1,2] Nevertheless, in both Europe and North America, the incidence

Disclosure Statement: We have no relevant disclosures.
Division of Gastroenterology, Department of Medicine Icahn School of Medicine at Mount Sinai, One Gustave Levy Place, Box 1069, New York, NY 10029, USA
* Corresponding author.
E-mail address: Michelle.Kim@mountsinai.org

of PNETs is rising.[3] Data from the Surveillance, Epidemiology, and End-Results Program suggest an incidence of 0.43/100,000 person-years today, compared with 0.17 in the 1970s.[2,3] This increase may be due to advances in diagnostic imaging and increased utilization of these technologies. Interestingly, autopsy studies have reported a widely varied incidence from 0.07% to as high as 10%, suggesting that many of these tumors are clinically silent and often go undiagnosed.[3–5] Approximately 90% of PNETs diagnosed in the United States are nonfunctioning.[6] PNETs can present at any age; however, the incidence peaks in the sixth and seventh decades.[6] Not surprisingly, functional tumors present earlier than nonfunctional tumors (mean age 55 vs 59 years).[6]

SYNDROMIC ASSOCIATION

Although 90% of PNETs occur sporadically, these tumors are also well-recognized features of 4 familial syndromes: multiple endocrine neoplasia type I (MEN1), von Hippel-Lindau syndrome (VHL), neurofibromatosis type 1 (NF1), and tuberous sclerosis complex (TSC).[7,8] Each of these syndromes is inherited in an autosomal dominant pattern, and the causative genes are *MEN1*, *VHL*, *NF1*, and *TSC1/2*, respectively. Whereas most patients (80%–100%) with *MEN1* develop PNET, the frequency is much lower among the 3 other syndromes. Among patients with VHL, NF1, and TSC, 10% to 17%, 0% to 10% (almost all duodenal somatostatinomas), and fewer than 1%, respectively, develop PNETs.[9] In general, PNETs that arise in the background of a familial syndrome tend to follow a more indolent course than sporadic tumors.

Multiple Endocrine Neoplasia Type I

MEN1 is characterized by PNETs in association with pituitary and parathyroid tumors. Almost all patients with MEN1 (>95%) will develop a PNET during their lifetime, although most of these will be nonfunctioning "micro-adenomas" (smaller than 0.5 cm) that are typically multifocal.[7,10,11] Fewer than 15% of these nonfunctioning tumors will be large enough to be symptomatic.[10] Functioning PNETs that are symptomatic occur in between 20% and 70% of patients with MEN1, with approximately 55% of these patients presenting with Zollinger-Ellison (ZE) syndrome due to an underlying gastrinoma, and 20% presenting with symptoms from an insulinoma.[7,8,10] Other functioning PNETs, such as VIPoma, glucagonoma, and somatostatinoma occur in fewer than 3% of patients with MEN1.[12] The management of patients with MEN1 with PNETs is of particular significance, as PNETs are the leading cause (40%) of disease-specific mortality among patients with MEN1.[13,14] Furthermore, the mean age of death among patients with MEN1 with PNETS is 55 years, which is lower than that of both the general population and patients with non-MEN1 PNETs.[14]

Von Hippel-Lindau Syndrome

Although pancreatic lesions are common in VHL, only 10% to 17% of patients with VHL develop PNETs.[7,8] Furthermore, almost all VHL-associated PNETs are nonfunctioning. The mean age of diagnosis of PNETs is 29 to 38 years, and unlike MEN1, most of these lesions are solitary as opposed to multifocal.[8]

CLASSIFICATION AND STAGING

Originally referred to as islet cell tumors, PNETs were renamed as such in 2010 by the World Health Organization (WHO). Over the past 10 years, groups such as WHO, American Joint Committee on Cancer (AJCC), and the European Neuroendocrine

Tumor Society (ENETS) have proposed formal staging systems for PNETs. All systems make a basic distinction between well-differentiated tumors, which tend to be more indolent, and poorly differentiated tumors, which tend to behave more aggressively.

The 2010 WHO classification of PNETs is based on the proliferative index of the tumor as measured by the Ki-67 index and mitotic count (**Table 1**).[15] This classification separates well-differentiated lesions into low-grade (G1) and intermediate-grade (G2) NETs, whereas all poorly differentiated lesions (G3) are labeled as neuroendocrine carcinomas.

With regard to staging, WHO endorses staging NETs based on the TNM classification; however, the AJCC manual and ENETS differ in their use of the TNM criteria. Whereas the AJCC manual stages PNETS using the same system developed for pancreatic adenocarcinoma, the ENETS proposal is modified specifically for PNETs and incorporates a different T-stage definition. The AJCC and ENETS staging systems are summarized in **Tables 2** and **3**.[16,17]

Although both the AJCC and the ENETS staging systems appear to be independent predictors of survival among patients with PNETs,[18–20] one large European cohort study found the ENETS system to provide more equally populated risk groups and more accurate predictive ability.[21]

PATHOPHYSIOLOGIC MECHANISMS

Although functioning PNETs may secrete hormones that are associated with the endocrine pancreas (islets of Langerhans), recent investigation has shown that PNETs actually arise from pluripotent stem cells of the exocrine (acinar/ductal) pancreas. These pluripotent cells then develop into atypical accumulations with both an exocrine and endocrine phenotype.[22] The most common driver mutations implicated in PNET tumorigenesis are *MEN1*, *DAXX/ATRX*, and mammalian target of Rapamycin (*mTOR*), found in 44%, 43%, and 14% of PNETs, respectively.[23]

MEN1 is a tumor suppressor gene that codes for the protein Menin. Loss of function of the *MEN1* gene may be inherited in an autosomal dominant fashion (*MEN1* syndrome) or be acquired as a sporadic mutation.[24] Regardless, mutation of *MEN1* is thought to be a proximal event in PNET tumorigenesis. *DAXX* and *ATRX* function together as a dimer and are involved in chromatin remodeling and stabilization.[25] Specifically, these proteins are associated with abnormal telomeres through a telomerase-independent telomere maintenance mechanism named ALT (alternative lengthening of telomeres).[26] Loss of *DAXX* or *ATRX* appears to result in reduced

Table 1 2010 WHO grading system for PNETs				
Differentiation	**Grade**	**Ki-67 Index**	**Mitotic Count**	**Nomenclature**

Well
  differentiated
	Low (G1)	<3%	<2 per 10 HPF	Neuroendocrine tumor,
				  grade 1

	Intermediate
	  (G2)
		3%–20%	2–20 per 10 HPF	Neuroendocrine tumor,
				  grade 2

Poorly differentiated	High (G3)	>20%	>20 per 10 HPF	Neuroendocrine carcinoma

Abbreviations: HPF, high-power field; WHO, World Health Organization.

Data from Bosnan FT, Carneiro F, Hruban RH, et al. WHO classification of tumours of the digestive system. Lyon (France): International Agency for Research on Cancer; 2010; and Klimstra DS, Modlin IR, Coppola D, et al. The pathologic classification of neuroendocrine tumors: a review of nomenclature, grading, and staging systems. Pancreas 2010;39(6):707–12.

Table 2
American Joint Committee on Cancer staging system for pancreatic cancer (used for both endocrine and exocrine tumors)

Stage	Tumor	Node	Metastasis	Description
1A	T1	N0	M0	Tumor limited to pancreas and size <2 cm
1B	T2	N0	M0	Tumor limited to pancreas and size >2 cm
IIA	T3	N0	M0	Tumor extends beyond pancreas but without involvement of the celiac axis of the superior mesenteric artery
IIB	T1–T3	N1	M0	Any tumor without artery involvement that has regional lymph node metastases
III	T4	Any N	M0	Tumor involves the celiac axis of the superior mesenteric artery
IV	Any T	Any N	M1	Any tumor with distant metastases

Data from Exocrine and endocrine pancreas. AJCC cancer staging manual. New York: Springer; 2010. p. 241–9.

time of relapse-free and tumor-associated survival, and may signify a more aggressive subtype of PNET.[27] The *mTOR* pathway is involved in cell survival and proliferation.[24] Abnormal activation of *mTOR* is common in patients with PNETs, and *mTOR* inhibitors are a current focus of targeted molecular therapy.[28–30]

CLINICAL PRESENTATION

The clinical presentation of PNETs is frequently divided into 2 broad categories: functioning and nonfunctioning tumors. Functional tumors present with a defined clinical syndrome secondary to hormone hypersecretion. Functional PNETs included insulinomas, gastrinomas, glucagonomas, VIPomas, and somatostatinomas. Nonfunctional tumors, which compromise 60% to 90% of all PNETs, do not present with symptoms related to hormone hypersecretion, although in some cases circulating hormone levels may be elevated nonetheless.[6,31,32]

Functional Tumors

Functional tumors represent the minority of PNETs, and the presenting symptoms depend on the hormone that is overproduced. Insulinomas are the most common

Table 3
European Neuroendocrine Tumor Society staging system for pancreatic neuroendocrine tumors

Stage	Tumor	Node	Metastasis	Description
I	T1	N0	M0	Tumor limited to the pancreas and size <2 cm
IIA	T2	N0	M0	Tumor limited to the pancreas and size 2–4 cm
IIB	T3	N0	M0	Tumor limited to the pancreas and size >4 cm or invading duodenum or bile duct
IIIA	T4	N0	M0	Tumor invading adjacent organs
IIIB	Any T	N1	M0	Any tumor that has regional lymph node metastases
IV	Any T	Any N	M1	Any tumor with distant metastases

Data from Rindi G, Klöppel G, Alhman H, et al. TNM staging of foregut (neuro)endocrine tumors: a consensus proposal including a grading system. Virchows Arch Int J Pathol 2006;449(4):395–401.

symptomatic PNET.[32,33] The Whipple triad is the diagnostic hallmark of insulinomas, which consists of documented hypoglycemia (plasma glucose <50 mg/dL), neuroglycopenic symptoms (confusion, visual change, diaphoresis, tremulousness), and rapid reversal of symptoms with administration of glucose.[34,35] Approximately 90% of patients exhibit the Whipple triad at the time of diagnosis.[35] Patients generally present in the fifth decade, with a higher incidence in men.[35] Gastrinomas are the second most common functional PNET.[32,33] Ectopic pancreatic or duodenal gastrin hypersecretion leads to symptoms of ZE syndrome, which are reflux, refractory peptic ulcer disease, and secretory diarrhea.[36] Glucagonomas, somatostatinomas, and VIPomas are rare and represent fewer than 10% of all functional PNETs.[7] The most common presenting symptom of glucagonoma is a classic rash, migratory necrolytic erythema, which is present in 52% of patients.[37] Surprisingly, diabetes develops in only 20% of patients before glucagonoma diagnosis.[37] Symptoms of glucagonoma are often summarized as the "4Ds": dermatitis, diabetes, depression, and deep vein thrombosis.[37] VIPomas often present with large-volume, watery diarrhea that is secretory in nature and may lead to dehydration and hypokalemia. Excess VIP secretion also may lead to flushing and electrolyte abnormalities, such as hyperglycemia, hypercalcemia, and hypochlorydria.[38,39] Somatostatinomas comprise fewer than 5% of PNETs, and are characterized by the clinical syndrome of diabetes mellitus, gallbladder disease, diarrhea, weight loss, and steatorrhea.[38,40] Nevertheless, it is exceedingly rare for patients to present with all of these features. In most cases, somatostatinomas are diagnosed by chance after a gastrointestinal NET demonstrates immunohistochemical staining for somastostatinlike immunoreactivity.[38,40]

Nonfunctional Tumors

Nonfunctional tumors represent 60% to 90% of all PNETs. As they do not present clinically with a hormonal syndrome, nonfunctional PNETs are often diagnosed later in the course of disease when they present with symptoms of compression or metastatic disease.[40] The most common presenting symptoms of nonfunctional PNETs are abdominal pain, weight loss, anorexia, and nausea. Patients may also infrequently present with obstructive jaundice, mimicking the presentation of pancreatic adenocarcinoma.

DIAGNOSTIC EVALUATION
Laboratory Evaluation

When patients present with clinical syndromes suspicious for PNETs, elevated levels of the hormone in question generally confirm the diagnosis. Glucagonoma, VIPoma, and somatostatinoma are associated with elevated serum levels of glucagon, VIP, and somatostatin, respectively. Insulinoma is diagnosed by measuring elevated serum insulin levels in the setting of hypoglycemia, which is often done after a prolonged, 48-hour to 72-hour fast.[35] Plasma glucose, C-peptide, and proinsulin also should be measured to rule out surreptitious insulin use.[35,40] Gastrinoma is associated with an elevated gastrin level in 99% of cases; however, this finding may be nonspecific. Patients with hypochlorhydria from atrophic gastritis/pernicious anemia, chronic *Helicobacter pylori* infection, or those on proton-pump inhibitors (PPIs) may also have physiologically elevated levels of gastrin.[36] As such, inappropriately elevated gastrin levels such as those associated with gastrinoma/ZE syndrome often require confirmation with a secretin stimulation test, which has a sensitivity of 94% and a specificity of 100%. PPIs should be stopped for a week before these tests.[41]

Several tumor markers have been studied with regard to PNETs. The most frequently used is chromogranin A (CgA), which is an acidic glycoprotein that is produced and excreted by granules within NETs.[42] CgA at a cutoff of 60.7 ng/mL has a sensitivity of 77% and a specificity of 56% for the diagnosis of PNETs. However, more recent analysis suggests that when insulinomas (which do not produce as much CgA) are excluded, a cutoff of 74 ng/mL has a specificity of as high as 91%.[43,44] A nomogram has recently been proposed to predict tumor burden, evaluate response, and predict survival for patients with well-differentiated PNETs and liver metastases based on CgA levels.[42] Other tumor markers proposed include pancreatic polypeptide and neuron specific enolase; however, their use in routine clinical practice remains less well defined.[45] Like CgA, all currently available biomarkers suffer from significant false-positive results.

Imaging

Several imaging modalities exist to aid the clinician in the localization and staging of PNETs. Computed tomography (CT), MRI, endoscopic ultrasound (EUS), somatostatin-receptor scintigraphy (SRS), and functional PET (fPET) are all commonly used in clinical practice. Arterial stimulation with venous sampling is a technique reserved for functional tumors that cannot be located with conventional techniques.

Computed tomography

CT scans are readily available, noninvasive tests often used in the diagnosis and staging of PNETs. PNETs are highly vascular lesions best appreciated with triple phase-contrast studies, as they enhance during the arterial phase with washout during the portal venous phase.[46] The sensitivity of CT scan for detecting PNETs ranges from 63% to 82% and the specificity ranges from 85% to 100%.[47] Two particular limitations of CT are the detection of lesions smaller than 2 cm and the detection of insulinomas. For these lesions, EUS is the imaging modality of choice.[48] The enhancement characteristics of a PNET on CT may also have prognostic value, as lesions that hypoenhance on CT scan tend to have worse overall survival than lesions that are isoenhancing or hyperenhancing (5-year survival 54% vs 89% vs 93%).[49]

MRI

MRI is frequently a modality of choice to evaluate pancreatic disease. The sensitivity of MRI for the detection of PNETs ranges from 85% to 100%, with a specificity from 75% to 100%.[47] Similar to CT, MRIs are best appreciated in the late arterial enhancement phase, and the signal is low in T1-weighted images and high in T2-weighted images. Specific MRI characteristics also may have prognostic value, as a study of 18 patients demonstrated that the apparent diffusion coefficient in diffusion-weighted MRI correlated with the Ki-67 labeling index.[50]

Endoscopic ultrasound

EUS is increasingly used in the evaluation of PNETs (**Fig. 1**). By combining endoscopy and ultrasound, EUS is not only able to localize and stage PNETs, but also to confirm and, in rare cases, treat disease.[51] EUS-guided fine-needle aspiration (EUS-FNA) is a reliable means of obtaining tissue for diagnosis, and EUS-guided injection of ablative agents, such as ethanol, has proven successful in the treatment of insulinomas in case reports.[52] EUS is superior to CT in the detection of smaller lesions, and can visualize PNETs as small as 2 to 5 mm.[48,51,53] Furthermore, EUS is particularly useful in the detection of insulinomas that are often multifocal, and may lack somatostatin receptors and are consequently not well visualized on SRS.[51,54] Limitations of EUS for the detection of PNETs include lesions in the pancreatic tail; this technique is also highly operator dependent.[51,55] Overall, the sensitivity and specificity for EUS in the detection of PNETs ranges from 82% to 93% and 92% to 95%.[51,53,56]

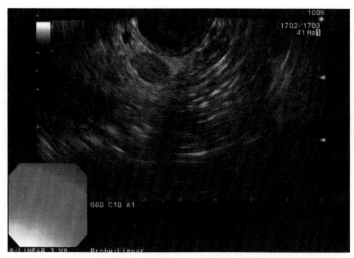

Fig. 1. EUS image of well-circumscribed 10.1 × 8.0-mm hypoechoic pancreatic head mass with peripheral enhancement consistent with NET. Pathology revealed well-differentiated, low-grade (G1) PNET. (*Courtesy of* Michelle Kang Kim, MD, PhD, New York, NY.)

Somatostatin-receptor scintigraphy

Similar to MRI, SRS is often used to localize PNETs when traditional cross-sectional imaging fails. SRS uses radiolabeled somatostatin analogues that bind to receptors expressed by the PNET.[47] Hence, lesions with few somatostatin receptors, such as insulinomas, are often missed with this technique. The standard method of performing SRS is with injection of 111In-DTPA-octreotide (OctreoScan).[57] SRS is particularly useful in assessing the burden of extrapancreatic metastatic disease, and also should be routinely performed to assess the somatostatin receptor status before treatment with somatostatin analogues. Overall, the sensitivity of SRS to detect gastrinomas, VIPomas, glucagonomas, and nonfunctioning PNETs ranges from 75% to 100%; however, for insulinomas, the sensitivity falls to 50% to 60%.[47,58]

PET

The role of PET scanning in the detection and staging of PNETs is evolving. Although traditional PET imaging with 18F-Fluorodeoxyglucose (FDG) is not useful for most PNETs, the emerging use of PET imaging with 68Ga-labeled somatostatin analogues and hybrid imaging with PET/CT have proven useful.[47] In a recent study of 23 PNETs, the diagnostic sensitivity of PET/CT with the somatostatin analogue 11-C-5-HTP was 96%, compared with 46%, 77%, and 68% for SRS, SRS/CT, and CT alone, respectively. However, because of limited availability of functional tracers, these new PET techniques are more widely available in Europe, and less routinely performed in North America. As such, functional and hybrid PET is generally reserved for cases in which conventional techniques fail or show contradictory results.[47]

TREATMENT

In general, surgery remains the cornerstone of treatment for PNETs and is the only curative option. Sporadic, nonmetastatic disease should be resected regardless of functional status. Depending on the location of the lesion, options include enucleation, central pancreatectomy, pancreaticoduodenectomy, and distal pancreatectomy.

Metastatic disease requires a multidisciplinary approach. Isolated liver metastases are treated aggressively with either surgery or local ablative or embolic therapies. For widespread metastatic disease, surgery remains an option provided that at least 90% of the tumor burden can be resected. The approach to nonresectable disease is based on the degree of differentiation of the lesion. Well-differentiated (G1 or G2) lesions are indolent and therapy is focused on symptom control. Options include somatostatin analogues, systemic chemotherapy, targeted molecular therapy, and peptide receptor radiotherapy. Poorly differentiated (G3) lesions respond well to chemotherapy but are associated with a more rapid deterioration and worse survival. The National Comprehensive Cancer Network has recently published clinical practice guidelines on the evaluation and treatment of PNETs.[59]

Surgery

Surgical resection remains the treatment of choice for sporadic, nonmetastatic disease; however, among patients with PNETs associated with a genetic syndrome, such as MEN1, VHL, NF1, or TSC, the role of surgery is more controversial.

Sporadic lesions

As mentioned previously, approximately 90% of PNETs are sporadic. For these lesions, surgery is the treatment of choice. Pancreaticoduodenectomy, distal pancreatectomy, and more parenchymal-preserving procedures, such as enucleation and central pancreatectomy, have all been used to treat PNETs. The choice of technique relies on several factors, including location of the lesion, malignant potential, functional status, and the presence of distant metastases. Although surgery may be performed for curative intent (as in the case of solitary, sporadic lesions), there is also a role for palliative debulking of the metastatic burden of PNETs, especially in the presence of functional tumors causing symptoms of hormonal excess.

Enucleation Pancreatic enucleation is a parenchymal-sparing procedure that results in much lower rates of endocrine and exocrine insufficiency than traditional pancreatic resection.[60–62] Previously, this procedure was reserved for small, low-grade PNETs; however, more recently enucleation is being considered as an alternative to standard resection in carefully selected patients.[63,64] One major limitation of this procedure is that it does not allow for adequate lymph node sampling, which may limit the potential of complete oncological resection in certain patients.[40] Nevertheless, comparable data are now emerging suggesting that enucleation should be the procedure of choice for small benign and premalignant lesions when technically appropriate.[63] A recent meta-analysis of 13 studies comprising 1101 patients found that compared with standard resection for small pancreatic lesions, enucleation was a shorter procedure that resulted in less blood loss and less pancreatic insufficiency despite comparable rates of mortality and complications. The most common complication associated with this procedure, pancreatic fistula, however, was higher in the enucleation group (odds ratio 1.99, confidence interval [CI] 1.2–3.4, $P<.01$).[62] Nevertheless, pancreatic fistulae that result from enucleation tend to be less severe than those following standard resection.[64] With regard to long-term survival, 5-year and 10-year survival appears no different between enucleation and standard resection.[63,64]

Central pancreatectomy Central pancreatectomy is another parenchymal-preserving procedure that may be indicated for lesions in the pancreatic neck or body, close to the pancreatic duct.[40] During this procedure, the pancreatic neck is divided, the tumor is excised, and pancreatico-jejunal or pancreatico-gastric anastomoses are created.[65] Similar to enucleation, central pancreatectomies have been increasingly performed in recent years.[66] Furthermore, compared with pancreaticoduodenectomy or distal pancreatectomy, central pancreatectomy is also associated with decreased operative time, less blood loss, and improved endocrine/exocrine function postoperatively with no difference in mortality.[67–72] Central pancreatectomy is technically challenging and traditionally performed open; however, recent series suggest promising results from laparoscopic and robot-assisted approaches.[73–75] Because central pancreatectomy does not allow access to adequate lymph node sampling, certain groups recommend it only for cases that would otherwise be appropriate for enucleation, but are not amenable due to location deep in the pancreatic parenchyma.[40]

Pancreaticoduodenectomy and distal pancreatectomy Pancreaticoduodenectomy and distal pancreatectomy are the more traditional surgical approaches to PNETs. Pancreaticoduodenectomy is indicated for lesions in the head of the pancreas, whereas distal pancreatectomy is used for lesions in the body or tail of the pancreas. Distal pancreatectomy may or may not be performed with concurrent splenectomy. Although splenic preservation is associated with decreased risk of infectious and severe complications, it is often reserved for more benign lesions like insulinomas, in which risk of malignancy is low and adequate lymph node harvest is less important.[40,76]

Treatment of hepatic metastases The surgical approach to metastatic disease divides patients into 2 categories: those with potentially resectable disease (often isolated liver metastases), and those with more extensive, unresectable disease. In general, the approach to patients with potentially resectable disease is aggressive. For isolated liver metastases, partial hepatectomy and less invasive methods, such as transarterial chemoembolization (TACE), radiofrequency ablation (RFA), yttrium-90 radioembolization (RE), cryotherapy, and microwave coagulation have all been used with varying degrees of success. An aggressive surgical approach for metastatic and locally advanced tumors is associated with increased long-term survival.[77,78]

Among patients with advanced PNETs and a large metastatic burden, surgery also may be considered even if complete resection is not possible. Although recurrence is expected, debulking is associated with improved symptom control and prolonged survival.[79–82] A recent retrospective study of 72 patients with nonfunctioning metastatic PNETs found a 1-year and 5-year disease-free survival rate of 58.1% and 3.5% for patients who underwent greater than 90% debulking of the tumor burden, similar to 53.7% and 10.7% for those who underwent complete resection.[83] With regard to symptom control, a separate series of 170 patients who underwent major debulking of hepatic metastases achieved a 96% rate of partial or complete response of symptoms, although this number included both ileal carcinoids and PNETs.[80] This improvement in symptom control may justify the high rate of recurrence of 88%, and the general consensus is that there is a role for palliative debulking as long as 90% of the disease burden can be resected.[80]

Multiple Endocrine Neoplasia Type I–Associated Lesions

The role of surgery for PNETs associated with MEN1 is less well defined, particularly for gastrinomas. For small gastrinomas, a prospective study of 81 patients with MEN1-associated gastrinomas found that patients with tumors smaller than 2.5 cm who did not undergo surgical resection had equivalent 15-year survival to those patients with tumors larger than 2.5 cm who did have surgery (89%–100%).[84] Hence, these small lesions can likely be observed without exposing the patient to the morbidity and mortality of pancreatic resection. For MEN1-associated gastrinomas larger than 2.5 cm, resection of solitary pancreatic lesions has been associated with improved long-term survival.[85] However, because MEN1-associated gastrinomas are often multiple and may be located in the duodenum, complete surgical resection may necessitate a formal pancreaticoduodenectomy. In these cases, expert opinion differs regarding medical versus surgical management.[86]

Insulinomas, glucagonomas, VIPomas, and somatostatinomas that arise in the background of MEN1 should be resected, as malignant PNETs constitute the leading cause of death among patients with MEN1.[14] For insulinomas, those associated with MEN1 are often multiple, small, and may evade conventional localization techniques. Hence, although these lesions should be resected, no definitive consensus exists regarding the optimal technique. Given that local resection has a high chance of failure, some advocate subtotal pancreatectomy with enucleation of lesions in the head of the pancreas.[87]

For nonfunctioning PNETs associated with MEN1, current guidelines suggest conservative management of lesions smaller than 1 cm, and resection of lesions larger than 2 cm or those that display rapid growth such as doubling in size over a 3-month to 6-month period.[86,88,89] Lesions 1 to 2 cm in size may be managed conservatively or surgically.[86]

Systemic Therapy

Although the only curative treatment for PNETs is surgery, several medical therapies exist for those with unresectable metastatic disease resulting in tumor bulk or hormonal excess. Well-differentiated and poorly differentiated PNETs respond differently to medical management, and therefore should be approached differently.

Well-differentiated pancreatic neuroendocrine tumors

Well-differentiated PNETs are either low-grade (G1) or intermediate-grade (G2) NETs. These tumors are more indolent, and medical management is generally focused on symptom control. For functioning tumors, initial therapy includes treating the manifestations of hormonal excess by using somatastatin analogues (SSAs) when appropriate. Systemic chemotherapy, targeted molecular therapy, and peptide receptor radiotherapy may be used for refractory disease and nonfunctioning tumors.

Hormonal excess and somatostatin analogues Conventional treatment of symptoms should be used whenever appropriate. For example, gastrinomas should be treated with high-dose PPI therapy, and insulinomas should be treated with carbohydrates and diazoxide. For refractory cases and other PNETs like VIPomas, somatostatinomas, and glucagonomas,[39,90] SSAs, such as octreotide or lanreotide, may be used. SSAs bind to somatostatin receptors expressed by most NETs and subsequently reduce the secretion of hormonally active peptides.[91] SSAs are generally less useful in insulinomas, as far fewer of these tumors express the somatostatin receptor.[51,54] Furthermore, symptoms of hypoglycemia may transiently worsen with concurrent suppression of glucagon secretion.

In addition to controlling the symptoms of hormonal excess, SSAs may also limit tumor growth. Most recently, a multinational study of well-differentiated and moderately differentiated metastatic enteropancreatic NETs comparing lanreotide with placebo found significantly improved progression-free survival for patients taking lanreotide (65.1% vs 33.0% at 24 months, hazard ratio (HR) 0.47, 95% CI 0.30–0.73). This result is consistent with previous studies examining tumor regression with SSAs in gastropancreatic NETs.[92–95] SSAs are generally well-tolerated, with the most common side effects being diarrhea/loose stools from pancreatic insufficiency, abdominal discomfort, nausea, and the development of gallstones.[96]

Chemotherapy Several chemotherapeutic regimens have been used to control the metastatic burden of PNETs. The initial standard therapy was with streptozocin-based regimens, but side effects, such as kidney injury, hair loss, and nausea, have limited the widespread adoption of such treatments. Instead, temozolomide and oxaliplatin-containing regimens are more often used. Temozolomide is an oral alkylating agent whose efficacy appears to be dependent on expression of the DNA repair enzyme O(6)-methylguanine-DNA methyltransferase (MGMT).[97,98] PNETs deficient in MGMT respond better to temozolomide-based therapy than those with intact expression.[97,98] Oxaliplatin is a platinum-based agent that when combined with capecitabine has shown efficacy in the treatment of well-differentiated NETs after progression with somatostatin analogues.[99]

Targeted molecular therapies Targeted molecular therapies for PNETs include those that target the vascular endothelial growth factor (VEGF) and mTOR pathways. Tyrosine kinase inhibitors, such as sunitinib, sorafenib, and pazopanib, as well as the direct VEGF blocker bevacizumab work via the VEGF pathway. Everolimus and temsirolimus inhibit the mTOR pathway.

Tyrosine kinase inhibitors Sunitinib is currently the only tyrosine kinase inhibitor approved by the Food and Drug Administration (FDA) for the treatment of unresectable, well-differentiated PNETs. Sunitinib is an orally available medication that targets the VEGF receptor pathway. A large randomized, phase III trial reported a median progression-free survival of 11.4 months for patients treated with sunitinib versus 5.4 months for placebo (HR 0.42, 95% CI 0.25–0.66, $P<.001$).[100] Sorafenib and pazopanib, although not FDA approved, have also shown promise in the treatment of PNETs. In a phase II trial of unresectable gastropancreatic NETs, which included 43 PNETs, progression-free survival was reported in 60.8% of evaluable patients with PNET. However, 43% of patients experienced significant grade 3 or 4 toxicity.[101]

Mammalian target of Rapamycin inhibitors Everolimus was FDA approved in 2011 for the treatment of unresectable, locally advanced, or metastatic PNETs based primarily on data from 2 large, phase III trials. RADIANT-2 compared everolimus plus octreotide with placebo plus octreotide in 429 patients with advanced, functionally active NETs. Patients treated with everolimus plus octreotide had improved median progression-free survival (PFS) (16.4 vs 11.3 months, $P = .026$).[102] RADIANT-3 compared daily everolimus 10 mg with placebo in 410 patients specifically with PNETs. Similarly, the everolimus-treated patients had an increased median PFS compared with placebo (11.0 vs 4.6 months, $P<.001$).[103] Temsirolimus was evaluated in a phase II trial of 37 patients with advanced, progressive, neuroendocrine carcinoma[104]; however, only a modest intention-to-treat response rate of 5.6% was noted. Hence, further studies investigating the use of temsirolimus as monotherapy for advanced NETs were deferred.

Bevacizumab Bevacizumab is a monoclonal antibody to circulating VEGF-A that inhibits angiogenesis and is currently used to treat a number of different malignancies.[105] With regard to NET, bevacizumab has been studied in conjunction with several other therapies, including everolimus, temsirolimus, and FOLFOX, with promising results.[105–107] Nevertheless, it is not FDA approved for the treatment of PNET and its use remains investigational. An open-label, phase II study also combined bevacizumab with sorafenib; however, despite a median PFS of 12.4 months, 63% of patients experienced a grade 3 or 4 adverse reaction.[108]

Peptide receptor radiotherapy Peptide receptor radiotherapy (PRRT) remains an investigational procedure in the United States, despite extensive experience in Europe. PRRT couples radioactive isotopes, such as yttrium (^{90}Y) and lutetium (^{177}Lu), to SSAs to deliver targeted radiotherapy to NET cells.[40] Early results are promising. The largest series of yttrium-coupled octreotide (90Y-DOTA-TOC) comprising 1109 patients with metastatic gastropancreatic NETs and disease progression treated with a median of 2 cycles of therapy found 34% of patients achieved radiographic response, 15% had biochemical response, and 29.7% had symptomatic improvement. The median survival from diagnosis was 94.6 months and the rates of transient grade 3 or 4 toxicity or permanent grade 4 or 5 toxicity were 12% and 9%, respectively.[109] A second study of 504 patients treated with Lu-177 reported similar efficacy but a much lower toxicity rate of 3.6%.[110]

Poorly differentiated pancreatic neuroendocrine tumors

Poorly differentiated PNETs are high-grade (G3) tumors that are referred to as neuroendocrine carcinomas. In general, poorly differentiated NETs respond better to chemotherapy, but are associated with a more rapid deterioration and worse survival.[111] Platinum-based chemotherapeutic regimens such as cisplatin and etoposide have shown promise in these lesions; however, prognosis remains poor.[112–114] A study of 36 patients with either poorly differentiated NETs or a rapidly progressing clinical course treated with cisplatin/etoposide showed a radiographic response rate of 36%, but a median survival time of only 19 months.[113] Few data exist for second-line therapy, and no studies have looked at PNETs specifically. Furthermore, little is known about the potential role of targeted molecular therapies or peptide receptor radiotherapy among patients with poorly differentiated PNETs.

SUMMARY

Islet cell tumors of the pancreas, also known as PNETs, are rare tumors that are increasing in incidence in North America and Europe. Most PNETs are nonfunctioning and diagnosed incidentally. However, PNETs may also present with distinct clinical syndromes secondary to hormonal excess. In a minority of cases, PNETs arise in the background of known genetic syndromes such as MEN1 or VHL. Accurate localization and staging are essential to the management of PNETs, for which surgical resection remains the cornerstone of treatment provided that 90% of the tumor burden can be resected. For nonresectable well-differentiated lesions, SSAs, chemotherapy, targeted molecular therapy, and most recently PRRT are appropriate options that lead to increased survival. Unfortunately, the prognosis for poorly differentiated PNETs remains poor.

REFERENCES

1. Fesinmeyer MD, Austin MA, Li CI, et al. Differences in survival by histologic type of pancreatic cancer. Cancer Epidemiol Biomarkers Prev 2005;14(7):1766–73.
2. Lawrence B, Gustafsson BI, Chan A, et al. The epidemiology of gastroenteropancreatic neuroendocrine tumors. Endocrinol Metab Clin North Am 2011; 40(1):1–18.
3. Fraenkel M, Kim MK, Faggiano A, et al. Epidemiology of gastroenteropancreatic neuroendocrine tumours. Best Pract Res Clin Gastroenterol 2012;26(6): 691–703.
4. Halfdanarson TR, Rubin J, Farnell MB, et al. Pancreatic endocrine neoplasms: epidemiology and prognosis of pancreatic endocrine tumors. Endocr Relat Cancer 2008;15(2):409–27.

5. Information NC for B., Pike USNL of M 8600 R., MD B., Usa 20894. Clinical pathology of endocrine tumors of the pancreas. Analysis of autopsy cases. Available at: http://eresources.library.mssm.edu:2132/pubmed/2070707. Accessed August 1, 2015.

6. Halfdanarson TR, Rabe KG, Rubin J, et al. Pancreatic neuroendocrine tumors (PNETs): incidence, prognosis and recent trend toward improved survival. Ann Oncol 2008;19(10):1727–33.

7. de Wilde RF, Edil BH, Hruban RH, et al. Well-differentiated pancreatic neuroendocrine tumors: from genetics to therapy. Nat Rev Gastroenterol Hepatol 2012; 9(4):199–208.

8. Jensen RT, Berna MJ, Bingham DB, et al. Inherited pancreatic endocrine tumor syndromes: advances in molecular pathogenesis, diagnosis, management, and controversies. Cancer 2008;113(S7):1807–43.

9. Metz DC, Jensen RT. Gastrointestinal neuroendocrine tumors: pancreatic endocrine tumors. Gastroenterology 2008;135(5):1469–92.

10. Yates CJ, Newey PJ, Thakker RV. Challenges and controversies in management of pancreatic neuroendocrine tumours in patients with MEN1. Lancet Diabetes Endocrinol 2015;3(11):895–905.

11. Anlauf M, Schlenger R, Perren A, et al. Microadenomatosis of the endocrine pancreas in patients with and without the multiple endocrine neoplasia type 1 syndrome. Am J Surg Pathol 2006;30(5):560–74.

12. Lévy-Bohbot N, Merle C, Goudet P, et al. Prevalence, characteristics and prognosis of MEN 1-associated glucagonomas, VIPomas, and somatostatinomas: study from the GTE (Groupe des Tumeurs Endocrines) registry. Gastroenterol Clin Biol 2004;28(11):1075–81.

13. Dean PG, van Heerden JA, Farley DR, et al. Are patients with multiple endocrine neoplasia type I prone to premature death? World J Surg 2000;24(11):1437–41.

14. Ito T, Igarashi H, Uehara H, et al. Causes of death and prognostic factors in multiple endocrine neoplasia type 1: a prospective study: comparison of 106 MEN1/Zollinger-Ellison syndrome patients with 1613 literature MEN1 patients with or without pancreatic endocrine tumors. Medicine (Baltimore) 2013;92(3):135–81.

15. Bosnan FT, Carneiro F, Hruban RH, et al. WHO classification of tumours of the digestive system. Lyon (France): International Agency for Research on Cancer; 2010.

16. Rindi G, Klöppel G, Alhman H, et al. TNM staging of foregut (neuro)endocrine tumors: a consensus proposal including a grading system. Virchows Arch Int J Pathol 2006;449(4):395–401.

17. Exocrine and Endocrine Pancreas. AJCC cancer staging manual. New York: Springer; 2010. p. 241–9.

18. Strosberg JR, Cheema A, Weber JM, et al. Relapse-free survival in patients with nonmetastatic, surgically resected pancreatic neuroendocrine tumors: an analysis of the AJCC and ENETS staging classifications. Ann Surg 2012;256(2): 321–5.

19. Ellison TA, Wolfgang CL, Shi C, et al. A single institution's 26-year experience with nonfunctional pancreatic neuroendocrine tumors: a validation of current staging systems and a new prognostic nomogram. Ann Surg 2014;259(2): 204–12.

20. Liu T-C, Hamilton N, Hawkins W, et al. Comparison of WHO classifications (2004, 2010), the Hochwald grading system, and AJCC and ENETS staging systems in predicting prognosis in locoregional well-differentiated pancreatic neuroendocrine tumors. Am J Surg Pathol 2013;37(6):853–9.

21. Rindi G, Falconi M, Klersy C, et al. TNM staging of neoplasms of the endocrine pancreas: results from a large international cohort study. J Natl Cancer Inst 2012;104(10):764–77.

22. Vortmeyer AO, Huang S, Lubensky I, et al. Non-islet origin of pancreatic islet cell tumors. J Clin Endocrinol Metab 2004;89(4):1934–8.

23. Jiao Y, Shi C, Edil BH, et al. DAXX/ATRX, MEN1, and mTOR pathway genes are frequently altered in pancreatic neuroendocrine tumors. Science 2011; 331(6021):1199–203.

24. Zhang J, Francois R, Iyer R, et al. Current understanding of the molecular biology of pancreatic neuroendocrine tumors. J Natl Cancer Inst 2013; 105(14):1005–17.

25. Tang J, Wu S, Liu H, et al. A novel transcription regulatory complex containing death domain-associated protein and the ATR-X syndrome protein. J Biol Chem 2004;279(19):20369–77.

26. Heaphy CM, de Wilde RF, Jiao Y, et al. Altered telomeres in tumors with ATRX and DAXX mutations. Science 2011;333(6041):425.

27. Marinoni I, Kurrer AS, Vassella E, et al. Loss of DAXX and ATRX are associated with chromosome instability and reduced survival of patients with pancreatic neuroendocrine tumors. Gastroenterology 2014;146(2):453–60.e5.

28. Missiaglia E, Dalai I, Barbi S, et al. Pancreatic endocrine tumors: expression profiling evidences a role for AKT-mTOR pathway. J Clin Oncol 2010;28(2): 245–55.

29. Zhou C-F, Ji J, Yuan F, et al. mTOR activation in well differentiated pancreatic neuroendocrine tumors: a retrospective study on 34 cases. Hepatogastroenterology 2011;58(112):2140–3.

30. Chan J, Kulke M. Targeting the mTOR signaling pathway in neuroendocrine tumors. Curr Treat Options Oncol 2014;15(3):365–79.

31. Panzuto F, Nasoni S, Falconi M, et al. Prognostic factors and survival in endocrine tumor patients: comparison between gastrointestinal and pancreatic localization. Endocr Relat Cancer 2005;12(4):1083–92.

32. Zerbi A, Falconi M, Rindi G, et al. Clinicopathological features of pancreatic endocrine tumors: a prospective multicenter study in Italy of 297 sporadic cases. Am J Gastroenterol 2010;105(6):1421–9.

33. Ito T, Tanaka M, Sasano H, et al. Preliminary results of a Japanese nationwide survey of neuroendocrine gastrointestinal tumors. J Gastroenterol 2007;42(6): 497–500.

34. Tucker ON, Crotty PL, Conlon KC. The management of insulinoma. Br J Surg 2006;93(3):264–75.

35. Mehrabi A, Fischer L, Hafezi M, et al. A systematic review of localization, surgical treatment options, and outcome of insulinoma. Pancreas 2014;43(5):675–86.

36. Ito T, Igarashi H, Jensen RT. Zollinger–Ellison syndrome: recent advances and controversies. Curr Opin Gastroenterol 2013;29(6):650–61.

37. Kindmark H, Sundin A, Granberg D, et al. Endocrine pancreatic tumors with glucagon hypersecretion: a retrospective study of 23 cases during 20 years. Med Oncol 2007;24(3):330–7.

38. Ito T, Igarashi H, Jensen RT. Pancreatic neuroendocrine tumors: clinical features, diagnosis and medical treatment: advances. Best Pract Res Clin Gastroenterol 2012;26(6):737–53.

39. Nikou GC, Toubanakis C, Nikolaou P, et al. VIPomas: an update in diagnosis and management in a series of 11 patients. Hepatogastroenterology 2005;52(64): 1259–65.

40. McKenna LR, Edil BH. Update on pancreatic neuroendocrine tumors. Gland Surg 2014;3(4):258–75.
41. Berna MJ, Hoffmann KM, Long SH, et al. Serum gastrin in Zollinger-Ellison syndrome: II. Prospective study of gastrin provocative testing in 293 patients from the National Institutes of Health and comparison with 537 cases from the literature. Evaluation of diagnostic criteria, proposal of new criteria, and correlations with clinical and tumoral features. Medicine (Baltimore) 2006;85(6):331–64.
42. Han X, Zhang C, Tang M, et al. The value of serum chromogranin A as a predictor of tumor burden, therapeutic response, and nomogram-based survival in well-moderate nonfunctional pancreatic neuroendocrine tumors with liver metastases. Eur J Gastroenterol Hepatol 2015;27(5):527–35.
43. Paik WH, Ryu JK, Song BJ, et al. Clinical usefulness of plasma chromogranin a in pancreatic neuroendocrine neoplasm. J Korean Med Sci 2013;28(5):750–4.
44. Qiao X-W, Qiu L, Chen Y-J, et al. Chromogranin A is a reliable serum diagnostic biomarker for pancreatic neuroendocrine tumors but not for insulinomas. BMC Endocr Disord 2014;14:64.
45. Vinik AI, Silva MP, Woltering G, et al. Biochemical testing for neuroendocrine tumors. Pancreas 2009;38(8):876–89.
46. Paulson EK, McDermott VG, Keogan MT, et al. Carcinoid metastases to the liver: role of triple-phase helical CT. Radiology 1998;206(1):143–50.
47. Sundin A. Radiological and nuclear medicine imaging of gastroenteropancreatic neuroendocrine tumours. Best Pract Res Clin Gastroenterol 2012;26(6):803–18.
48. Khashab MA, Yong E, Lennon AM, et al. EUS is still superior to multidetector computerized tomography for detection of pancreatic neuroendocrine tumors. Gastrointest Endosc 2011;73(4):691–6.
49. Worhunsky DJ, Krampitz GW, Poullos PD, et al. Pancreatic neuroendocrine tumours: hypoenhancement on arterial phase computed tomography predicts biological aggressiveness. HPB (Oxford) 2014;16(4):304–11.
50. Wang Y, Chen ZE, Yaghmai V, et al. Diffusion-weighted MR imaging in pancreatic endocrine tumors correlated with histopathologic characteristics. J Magn Reson Imaging 2011;33(5):1071–9.
51. Kim MK. Endoscopic ultrasound in gastroenteropancreatic neuroendocrine tumors. Gut Liver 2012;6(4):405–10.
52. Jürgensen C, Schuppan D, Neser F, et al. EUS-guided alcohol ablation of an insulinoma. Gastrointest Endosc 2006;63(7):1059–62.
53. Rösch T, Lightdale CJ, Botet JF, et al. Localization of pancreatic endocrine tumors by endoscopic ultrasonography. N Engl J Med 1992;326(26):1721–6.
54. Sotoudehmanesh R, Hedayat A, Shirazian N, et al. Endoscopic ultrasonography (EUS) in the localization of insulinoma. Endocrine 2007;31(3):238–41.
55. Wani S, Coté GA, Keswani R, et al. Learning curves for EUS by using cumulative sum analysis: implications for American Society for Gastrointestinal Endoscopy recommendations for training. Gastrointest Endosc 2013;77(4):558–65.
56. Anderson MA, Carpenter S, Thompson NW, et al. Endoscopic ultrasound is highly accurate and directs management in patients with neuroendocrine tumors of the pancreas. Am J Gastroenterol 2000;95(9):2271–7.
57. Kwekkeboom DJ, Krenning EP, Scheidhauer K, et al. ENETS consensus guidelines for the standards of care in neuroendocrine tumors: somatostatin receptor imaging with (111)In-pentetreotide. Neuroendocrinology 2009;90(2):184–9.
58. de Herder WW, Kwekkeboom DJ, Valkema R, et al. Neuroendocrine tumors and somatostatin: imaging techniques. J Endocrinol Invest 2005;28(11 Suppl International):132–6.

59. Kulke MH, Shah MH, Benson AB, et al. Neuroendocrine tumors, version 1.2015. J Natl Compr Cancer Netw 2015;13(1):78–108.
60. Crippa S, Boninsegna L, Partelli S, et al. Parenchyma-sparing resections for pancreatic neoplasms. J Hepatobiliary Pancreat Sci 2010;17(6):782–7.
61. Hackert T, Hinz U, Fritz S, et al. Enucleation in pancreatic surgery: indications, technique, and outcome compared to standard pancreatic resections. Langenbecks Arch Surg 2011;396(8):1197–203.
62. Chua TC, Yang TX, Gill AJ, et al. Systematic review and meta-analysis of enucleation versus standardized resection for small pancreatic lesions. Ann Surg Oncol 2015. http://dx.doi.org/10.1245/s10434-015-4826-3.
63. Cauley CE, Pitt HA, Ziegler KM, et al. Pancreatic enucleation: improved outcomes compared to resection. J Gastrointest Surg 2012;16(7):1347–53.
64. Pitt SC, Pitt HA, Baker MS, et al. Small pancreatic and periampullary neuroendocrine tumors: resect or enucleate? J Gastrointest Surg 2009;13(9):1692–8.
65. Efron D. Central pancreatectomy with pancreaticogastrostomy for benign pancreatic pathology. J Gastrointest Surg 2004;8(5):532–8.
66. DiNorcia J, Lee MK, Reavey PL, et al. One hundred thirty resections for pancreatic neuroendocrine tumor: evaluating the impact of minimally invasive and parenchyma-sparing techniques. J Gastrointest Surg 2010;14(10):1536–46.
67. Crippa S, Bassi C, Warshaw AL, et al. Middle pancreatectomy: indications, short- and long-term operative outcomes. Ann Surg 2007;246(1):69–76.
68. Müller MW, Friess H, Kleeff J, et al. Middle segmental pancreatic resection: an option to treat benign pancreatic body lesions. Ann Surg 2006;244(6):909–18 [discussion: 918–20].
69. Hirono S, Tani M, Kawai M, et al. A central pancreatectomy for benign or low-grade malignant neoplasms. J Gastrointest Surg 2009;13(9):1659–65.
70. Sudo T, Murakami Y, Uemura K, et al. Middle pancreatectomy with pancreaticogastrostomy: a technique, operative outcomes, and long-term pancreatic function. J Surg Oncol 2010;101(1):61–5.
71. Shikano T, Nakao A, Kodera Y, et al. Middle pancreatectomy: safety and long-term results. Surgery 2010;147(1):21–9.
72. DiNorcia J, Ahmed L, Lee MK, et al. Better preservation of endocrine function after central versus distal pancreatectomy for mid-gland lesions. Surgery 2010;148(6):1247–54 [discussion: 1254–6].
73. Cheng K, Shen B, Peng C, et al. Initial experiences in robot-assisted middle pancreatectomy. HPB (Oxford) 2013;15(4):315–21.
74. Kuroki T, Eguchi S. Laparoscopic parenchyma-sparing pancreatectomy. J Hepatobiliary Pancreat Sci 2014;21(5):323–7.
75. Iacono C, Ruzzenente A, Bortolasi L, et al. Central pancreatectomy: the Dagradi Serio Iacono operation. Evolution of a surgical technique from the pioneers to the robotic approach. World J Gastroenterol 2014;20(42):15674–81.
76. Shoup M, Brennan MF, McWhite K, et al. The value of splenic preservation with distal pancreatectomy. Arch Surg 2002;137(2):164–8.
77. Kazanjian KK, Reber HA, Hines OJ. Resection of pancreatic neuroendocrine tumors: results of 70 cases. Arch Surg 2006;141(8):765–9 [discussion: 769–70].
78. Birnbaum DJ, Turrini O, Vigano L, et al. Surgical management of advanced pancreatic neuroendocrine tumors: short-term and long-term results from an international multi-institutional study. Ann Surg Oncol 2015;22(3):1000–7.
79. Norton JA, Kivlen M, Li M, et al. Morbidity and mortality of aggressive resection in patients with advanced neuroendocrine tumors. Arch Surg 2003;138(8):859–66.

80. Sarmiento JM, Heywood G, Rubin J, et al. Surgical treatment of neuroendocrine metastases to the liver: a plea for resection to increase survival. J Am Coll Surg 2003;197(1):29–37.
81. Dixon E, Pasieka JL. Functioning and nonfunctioning neuroendocrine tumors of the pancreas. Curr Opin Oncol 2007;19(1):30–5.
82. Chamberlain RS, Canes D, Brown KT, et al. Hepatic neuroendocrine metastases: does intervention alter outcomes? J Am Coll Surg 2000;190(4):432–45.
83. Cusati D, Zhang L, Harmsen WS, et al. Metastatic nonfunctioning pancreatic neuroendocrine carcinoma to liver: surgical treatment and outcomes. J Am Coll Surg 2012;215(1):117–24 [discussion: 124–5].
84. Norton JA, Alexander HR, Fraker DL, et al. Comparison of surgical results in patients with advanced and limited disease with multiple endocrine neoplasia type 1 and Zollinger-Ellison syndrome. Ann Surg 2001;234(4):495–505 [discussion 505–6].
85. Norton JA, Jensen RT. Role of surgery in Zollinger-Ellison syndrome. J Am Coll Surg 2007;205(4, Supplement):S34–7.
86. Sadowski SM, Triponez F. Management of pancreatic neuroendocrine tumors in patients with MEN 1. Gland Surg 2015;4(1):63–8.
87. Demeure MJ, Klonoff DC, Karam JH, et al. Insulinomas associated with multiple endocrine neoplasia type I: the need for a different surgical approach. Surgery 1991;110(6):998–1004 [discussion: 1004–5].
88. Triponez F, Goudet P, Dosseh D, et al. Is surgery beneficial for MEN1 patients with small (< or = 2 cm), nonfunctioning pancreaticoduodenal endocrine tumor? An analysis of 65 patients from the GTE. World J Surg 2006;30(5):654–62 [discussion: 663–4].
89. Kouvaraki MA, Shapiro SE, Cote GJ, et al. Management of pancreatic endocrine tumors in multiple endocrine neoplasia type 1. World J Surg 2006;30(5):643–53.
90. Angeletti S, Corleto VD, Schillaci O, et al. Use of the somatostatin analogue octreotide to localise and manage somatostatin-producing tumours. Gut 1998;42(6):792–4.
91. Reubi JC, Kvols LK, Waser B, et al. Detection of somatostatin receptors in surgical and percutaneous needle biopsy samples of carcinoids and islet cell carcinomas. Cancer Res 1990;50(18):5969–77.
92. Saltz L, Trochanowski B, Buckley M, et al. Octreotide as an antineoplastic agent in the treatment of functional and nonfunctional neuroendocrine tumors. Cancer 1993;72(1):244–8.
93. Arnold R, Trautmann ME, Creutzfeldt W, et al. Somatostatin analogue octreotide and inhibition of tumour growth in metastatic endocrine gastroenteropancreatic tumours. Gut 1996;38(3):430–8.
94. Ricci S, Antonuzzo A, Galli L, et al. Long-acting depot lanreotide in the treatment of patients with advanced neuroendocrine tumors. Am J Clin Oncol 2000;23(4):412–5.
95. Bianchi A, De Marinis L, Fusco A, et al. The treatment of neuroendocrine tumors with long-acting somatostatin analogs: a single center experience with lanreotide autogel. J Endocrinol Invest 2011;34(9):692–7.
96. Newman CB, Melmed S, Snyder PJ, et al. Safety and efficacy of long-term octreotide therapy of acromegaly: results of a multicenter trial in 103 patients–a clinical research center study. J Clin Endocrinol Metab 1995;80(9):2768–75.
97. Kulke MH, Hornick JL, Frauenhoffer C, et al. O6-methylguanine DNA methyltransferase deficiency and response to temozolomide-based therapy in patients with neuroendocrine tumors. Clin Cancer Res 2009;15(1):338–45.

98. Walter T, van Brakel B, Vercherat C, et al. O6-Methylguanine-DNA methyltransferase status in neuroendocrine tumours: prognostic relevance and association with response to alkylating agents. Br J Cancer 2015;112(3):523–31.
99. Bajetta E, Catena L, Procopio G, et al. Are capecitabine and oxaliplatin (XELOX) suitable treatments for progressing low-grade and high-grade neuroendocrine tumours? Cancer Chemother Pharmacol 2007;59(5):637–42.
100. Raymond E, Dahan L, Raoul J-L, et al. Sunitinib malate for the treatment of pancreatic neuroendocrine tumors. N Engl J Med 2011;364(6):501–13.
101. Hobday TJ, Rubin J, Holen K, et al. Mco44h, a phase II trial of sorafenib in patients (pts) with metastatic neuroendocrine tumors (NET): a phase II consortium (P2C) study. J Clin Oncol 2007;(25):S4504.
102. Pavel ME, Hainsworth JD, Baudin E, et al. Everolimus plus octreotide long-acting repeatable for the treatment of advanced neuroendocrine tumours associated with carcinoid syndrome (RADIANT-2): a randomised, placebo-controlled, phase 3 study. Lancet 2011;378(9808):2005–12.
103. Yao JC, Shah MH, Ito T, et al. Everolimus for advanced pancreatic neuroendocrine tumors. N Engl J Med 2011;364(6):514–23.
104. Duran I, Kortmansky J, Singh D, et al. A phase II clinical and pharmacodynamic study of temsirolimus in advanced neuroendocrine carcinomas. Br J Cancer 2006;95(9):1148–54.
105. Naraev BG, Strosberg JR, Halfdanarson TR. Current status and perspectives of targeted therapy in well-differentiated neuroendocrine tumors. Oncology 2012; 83(3):117–27.
106. Khagi S, Saif MW. Pancreatic neuroendocrine tumors: targeting the molecular basis of disease. Curr Opin Oncol 2015;27(1):38–43.
107. Yao JC, Phan AT, Hess K, et al. Perfusion computed tomography as functional biomarker in randomized run-in study of bevacizumab and everolimus in well-differentiated neuroendocrine tumors. Pancreas 2015;44(2):190–7.
108. Castellano D, Capdevila J, Sastre J, et al. Sorafenib and bevacizumab combination targeted therapy in advanced neuroendocrine tumour: a phase II study of Spanish Neuroendocrine Tumour Group (GETNE0801). Eur J Cancer 2013; 49(18):3780–7.
109. Imhof A, Brunner P, Marincek N, et al. Response, survival, and long-term toxicity after therapy with the radiolabeled somatostatin analogue [90Y-DOTA]-TOC in metastasized neuroendocrine cancers. J Clin Oncol 2011;29(17):2416–23.
110. Kwekkeboom DJ, de Herder WW, Kam BL, et al. Treatment with the radiolabeled somatostatin analog [177 Lu-DOTA 0,Tyr3]octreotate: toxicity, efficacy, and survival. J Clin Oncol 2008;26(13):2124–30.
111. Sorbye H, Welin S, Langer SW, et al. Predictive and prognostic factors for treatment and survival in 305 patients with advanced gastrointestinal neuroendocrine carcinoma (WHO G3): the NORDIC NEC study. Ann Oncol 2013;24(1): 152–60.
112. Moertel CG, Kvols LK, O'Connell MJ, et al. Treatment of neuroendocrine carcinomas with combined etoposide and cisplatin. Evidence of major therapeutic activity in the anaplastic variants of these neoplasms. Cancer 1991;68(2): 227–32.
113. Fjällskog ML, Granberg DP, Welin SL, et al. Treatment with cisplatin and etoposide in patients with neuroendocrine tumors. Cancer 2001;92(5):1101–7.
114. Mitry E, Baudin E, Ducreux M, et al. Treatment of poorly differentiated neuroendocrine tumours with etoposide and cisplatin. Br J Cancer 1999;81(8):1351–5.

Imaging of the Pancreas

Ming-ming Xu, MD, Amrita Sethi, MD*

KEYWORDS

- Contrast-enhanced harmonic endoscopic ultrasound • Endoscopic ultrasound
- Elastography • Intraductal pancreatic mucinous neoplasm
- Mucinous cystic neoplasm • Probe-based confocal endomicroscopy
- Serous cystic neoplasm

KEY POINTS

- Preoperative imaging of the pancreas has become a critical part of the evaluation, diagnosis, and staging of pancreatic cancer and other pancreatic neoplasms.
- Endoscopic ultrasound scan is associated with higher sensitivities for diagnosing pancreatic solid lesions and cystic lesions compared with cross-section imaging with MRI or multidetector computed tomography.
- New advances in endoscopic ultrasound scan enhancement with elastography and contrast enhancement may provide improvement in distinguishing malignant from benign inflammatory pancreatic diseases.

INTRODUCTION

Pancreatic mass lesions are highly concerning for pancreatic cancer, which remains highly fatal cancer and the fourth leading cause of cancer-related deaths. The American Cancer Society estimates 48,960 new cases of pancreatic cancer diagnosed in 2015 with an almost equal number of cancer-related deaths.[1] Preoperative imaging of the pancreas has become a critical part of the evaluation, diagnosis, and staging of pancreatic cancer and other pancreatic neoplasms. Early and accurate detection and staging of pancreatic neoplasms allows for curative resection in select patients, and avoidance of surgery in those who would not benefit and in whom further workup is indicated.

With the increased use of cross-sectional imaging, incidentally discovered pancreatic cysts have also become a common clinical problem. An estimated 15% of patients undergoing MRI of the abdomen are found to have a pancreatic cyst.[2] Although cystic neoplasms of the pancreas only account for 1% to 5% of all malignant

Disclosures: Boston Scientific-Consultant, Mauna Kea Technologies-travel reimbursement (A. Sethi).
Division of Digestive and Liver Disease, Columbia University Medical Center, 622 West 168th Street, New York, NY 10032, USA
* Corresponding author. 161 Fort Washington Avenue, Suite 852, Herbert Irving Pavilion, New York, NY 10032.
E-mail addresses: as3614@columbia.edu; as3614@cumc.columbia.edu

pancreatic neoplasms, they generate a substantial volume of subsequent imaging and procedures to differentiate between benign and malignant lesions. This imaging, in turn, has led to advances in radiologic and endoscopic-based imaging studies to better characterize the nature of these cysts. This report reviews the range of imaging tools currently available to evaluate pancreatic lesions, from solid tumors to pancreatic cysts. This article reviews noninvasive radiologic imaging and moves to the evolving role of endoscopic ultrasound scan (EUS) and the newer techniques of elastography and contrast-enhanced EUS. Finally, recent device innovations moving the field toward in vivo endoscopic microscopy of the pancreas are discussed.

RADIOLOGIC IMAGING OF THE PANCREAS
Solid Pancreatic Lesions

The most common etiology of a solid pancreatic tumor is adenocarcinoma, which accounts for 85% to 95% of all pancreatic tumors.[3] A few other malignant pancreatic neoplasms in the differential diagnosis of a solid pancreatic tumor have a generally more favorable prognosis compared with adenocarcinoma (**Box 1**). Noninvasive cross-sectional imaging of the pancreas remains the first-line imaging modality of choice in the evaluation of a pancreatic mass (**Table 1**). Cross-sectional studies can provide a general assessment of malignancy potential, resectability, presence of lymphadenopathy, and distant metastases.

Dual-phase multidetector computed tomography (MDCT) is an excellent initial imaging choice in the evaluation of pancreatic masses and is often referred to as *pancreatic protocol computed tomography* (CT). It provides 1-mm thick cross-sectional images of the pancreas with volume acquisition and allows for 3-dimensional reconstruction and vascular mapping in multiplanar views.[10] The dual contrast phase obtains images of the pancreatic parenchyma during the arterial phase and peripancreatic vasculature during the portal venous phase. Most pancreatic masses are hypoattenuating and best visualized during the portal venous phase, although certain neuroendocrine tumors and metastatic deposits to the pancreas can be hypervascular.[10] Signs used on MDCT to detect a small pancreatic mass even when no overt lesion is visible include concurrent biliary and pancreatic ductal dilation or "double duct" sign for pancreatic head tumors, subtle changes in the contour of the pancreas, or loss of perivascular fat planes.[11,12] In a head-to-head prospective comparison of the diagnostic yield of MDCT to EUS, DeWitt and colleagues[4] found MDCT to have lower sensitivity of overall cancer detection (86% vs 98% for EUS, $P = .01$), but MDCT was equivalent to EUS for tumor nodal staging. Although CT imaging overall has a high positive predictive value of more than 90% for tumor detection,[13,14] it is limited by poor detection of small tumors, critically those tumors in the early resectable stage, small hepatic metastases, and peritoneal implants.[15,16]

Box 1
Differential diagnosis of solid pancreatic tumors

Pancreatic adenocarcinoma

Pancreatic neuroendocrine tumor

Pancreatoblastoma

Pancreatic lymphoma

Solid pseudopapillary tumor

Table 1 Diagnostic yield of imaging modalities for pancreatic malignancy			
Imaging Modality	Sensitivity for Tumor Detection (%)	Specificity (%)	Accuracy of Tumor Nodal Staging (%)
CT	68–86	50–64	47–68
MRI	83–96	100	56–60
EUS	87–100	75–100	44–84

Data from Refs.[4–9]

On MRI, pancreatic tumors appear as a hypoenhancing lesion on T1-weighted images compared with the surrounding pancreatic parenchyma.[3] Overall, MRI sensitivity for tumor detection is similar to that of MDCT with reported ranges up to 90%.[17] However MRI may have an advantage of superior detection of smaller tumors and metastases, especially with the addition of newer techniques of diffusion-weighted MRI.[18,19] One distinct advantage of pancreatic MRI is the ability to obtain magnetic resonance cholangiopancreatography sequences to evaluate for pancreatic ductal dilation and biliary tract pathology, which has comparable diagnostic value for biliary obstruction to endoscopic retrograde cholangiopancreatography.[20,21]

Pancreatic Cysts

Cystic pancreatic neoplasms account for 1% to 5% of malignant pancreatic neoplasms, but they are increasingly recognized as an incidental finding during abdominal imaging studies obtained for other indications. Because the etiologies of pancreatic cysts encompass a wide range—from benign, inflammatory to malignant—determining the underlying etiology of the cyst is critical for prognostication and planning for either surgical resection or continued surveillance of lesions with low malignant potential (**Box 2**). Of the etiologies of cystic lesions, pseudocyst and serous cystadenoma are benign lesions with little to no malignant potential. Mucinous cystic neoplasm (MCN) is considered a premalignant lesion with a reported rate of malignant transformation of between 6% and 36%.[4,22–25] Intraductal papillary mucinous neoplasms (IPMN) have variable malignant potential depending on the subtype of IPMN with main-duct IPMN (MD-IPMN) having the highest malignant potential of between 57% and 92% in different series.[26–28]

Box 2 Differential diagnosis of cystic lesions of the pancreas
Serous cystadenoma
Mucinous cystic neoplasm
Intraductal papillary mucinous neoplasm
Pseudocyst
Cystic neuroendocrine tumor
Polycystic disease
Parasitic infection
Solid pseudopapillary neoplasm
Cystic degeneration of necrotic adenocarcinoma or metastases

In general, when an incidental cystic lesion is discovered, the radiologic imaging study of choice to further delineate cyst characteristics is MRI with magnetic resonance cholangiopancreatography because of MRI's superior soft tissue resolution compared with MDCT and the ability to evaluate the pancreatic duct and biliary tree.[29,30] MRI can identify pathognomonic features of the cyst subtypes, detect nodules, and main pancreatic duct involvement for risk stratification (**Table 2**). Retrospective studies show MRI accuracy in correctly classifying cysts as mucinous versus nonmucinous as 79% to 84%, but MRI performs poorly in diagnosing the specific subtype with an accuracy of only 44%.[30–32] However, MRI accuracy in predicting malignancy in a cystic lesion is reported to be 75%, comparable to EUS in one retrospective series.[33]

ENDOSCOPIC ULTRASOUND SCAN
Solid Pancreatic Mass

EUS is widely considered the most reliable and accurate test in the detection and diagnosis of pancreatic masses, including pancreatic cancer (**Fig. 1**).[34] Reported sensitivity of EUS in detection of pancreatic cancer is between 94% and 100%.[35–37] Compared with MDCT, EUS can detect between 13% and 14% of pancreatic cancers that were missed on MDCT.[4,37] In particular, EUS performs better with detection of tumors smaller than 20 mm where MRI and CT have higher miss rates.[38] For lymph node staging, EUS has an accuracy of 44% to 84%[4–6] with the lower accuracy attributed to variable appearance of metastatic lymph nodes and adenopathy that are obscured by the primary tumor and its associated inflammatory changes.[39] Current ultrasound criteria for malignant adenopathy include round, hypoechoic, lymph nodes with diameter greater than 1 cm with distinct margins. However, these features can be seen even in benign lymph nodes, and malignant nodes do not uniformly have all these

Table 2
Imaging (CT or MRI) features of pancreatic cystic neoplasms

Cyst Type	Clinical Features	Imaging Characteristics
Pseudocyst	Sequela of acute necrotizing pancreatitis, no sex predominance	Unilocular, encapsulated cyst with a well-defined wall
Serous cystadenoma	Older age, female predominance	Multilocular, microcystic appearance, central scar (seen in 30%) is pathognomonic
Mucinous cystic neoplasm	Sixth decade of life, almost all female	Multilocular, well encapsulated, smooth margins, preferentially in body or tail of pancreas, internal septations, peripheral calcification (16%) rare but specific for malignancy
SPEN	Young age, female predominant	Unilocular, encapsulated, can have solid and hemorrhagic components
IPMN	Older age, mild male predominance, often incidental finding	Any region of pancreas, MD-IPMN associated with pancreatic duct dilation >5 mm, dilated side branches seen in BD-IPMN

Abbreviations: BD-IPMN, branch duct intraductal papillary mucinous neoplasm; SPEN, Solid pseudopapillary neoplasm.

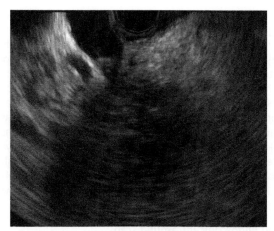

Fig. 1. EUS image of pancreatic adenocarcinoma. The hypoechoic mass seen in the head of the pancreas with bile duct obstruction represents typical EUS imaging of pancreatic adenocarcinomas.

features. The last component of cancer staging is an evaluation of vascular invasion. EUS sensitivity and specificity for vascular involvement is reported to be 56% to 87% and 89% to 97%, respectively.[5,7,40] EUS evaluation of the superior mesenteric vessels can be particularly difficult, as the course of these vessels through the uncinate and inferior head can be challenging to see.[41] Nevertheless, a retrospective analysis of Surveillance, Epidemiology, and End Results data found that patients who underwent EUS for pancreatic cancer were more likely to have earlier-stage disease, receive curative-intent surgery, and undergo chemotherapy and radiation therapy.[42] Overall, EUS was an independent predictor of improved survival in those who had it as part of their diagnosis or staging.[42]

Despite the overall reliability and utility of EUS in pancreatic imaging, it does have notable limitations. EUS can miss true pancreatic masses in the setting of chronic pancreatitis, at the site of the ventral/dorsal split of the pancreas, and when there are indwelling biliary or pancreatic stents causing acoustic shadowing.[43] EUS can also misdiagnose a pancreatic tumor in autoimmune pancreatitis, a well-known mimicker of pancreatic cancer that often presents with obstructive jaundice, abdominal pain, and a focal pancreatic head mass. Recently, 2 additional EUS-based imaging modalities, elastography and contrast-enhanced EUS, were studied with variable success in providing additional yield in the evaluation of pancreatic tumors, and some of the limitations of conventional EUS were addressed.

Elastography

Elastography refers to the measurement of relative tissue stiffness to differentiate benign and malignant pancreatic masses.[44] Malignant tissue is thought to have a harder consistency and thus has a different degree of compression compared with benign tissue. During EUS, real-time calculation of tissue elasticity can be performed using the natural arterial pulsations and respiratory movements as the source of pressure; the results are displayed in color superimposed onto conventional B-mode gray-scale scans.[45] Initial reports of the diagnostic accuracy of elastography showed sensitivity of near 100% in both malignant pancreatic mass and lymph nodes but low specificity caused by false-positive results of 67% for malignant lesions and 50% for lymph nodes.[45] Follow-up studies found inconsistent results, with one prospective study of 70 patients with undifferentiated pancreatic masses reporting much lower overall sensitivity of elastography of 41% for malignancy, specificity of 53%, and accuracy of only 45%.[46] Recent efforts to improve the reproducibility, accuracy, and clinical utility of elastography in pancreatic imaging have moved toward developing quantitative scoring systems for elastography to better delineate the relative differences in the elasticity of solid pancreatic masses.[47] Although performing elastography does not add significant time to an EUS examination, there are some limitations to adaptation of this technology. Elastography is not universally available as a built-in feature in all processors. Expensive software is required to supplement this feature into processors such as the Olympus ProSound F75. Furthermore, all endosonographers are not trained in elastography further limiting its availability. Special training in interpretation of elastography should be obtained, as varied interobserver agreement exists and can improve with experience[48] (**Fig. 2**).

Contrast-enhanced endoscopic ultrasound scan

Use of contrast-enhanced endosonography was initially introduced for ultrasound examinations of hepatic lesions in which microbubbles of inert gas were injected intravenously to enhance visualization of mass vascularity.[49] Similarly, contrast-enhanced EUS (CH-EUS) depends on the differential perfusion or enhancement pattern of pancreatic tumors to identify them, namely the hypovascular appearance of adenocarcinoma compared with the hypervascular appearance of pancreatic neuroendocrine tumor (NET) and isovascular appearance of the pancreatic parenchyma in chronic pancreatitis.[50] A meta-analysis of available data on CH-EUS with 1139 patients shows it has a pooled sensitivity of 94% for the diagnosis of pancreatic adenocarcinoma with specificity of 89%.[51] The meta-analysis included patients with chronic pancreatitis in whom conventional EUS is known to have poorer detection rates. Despite the promising data, the interpretation of CH-EUS images remains subjective, and there is a lack of data on the reproducibility of this novel technique outside of expert hands, thus limiting its widespread adoption. Furthermore, contrast agents are not currently approved or available in countries such as the United States (**Fig. 3**).

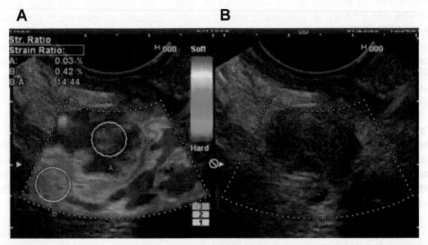

Fig. 2. EUS elastography. The area that appears blue (*A*) represents firmer tissue, consistent with neoplastic tissue compared with the green or more elastic tissue (*B*) of adjacent normal pancreas. (*Courtesy of* Francis G. Gress, MD, New York, NY.)

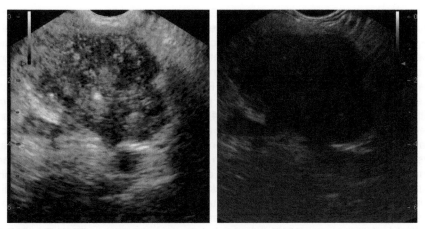

Fig. 3. Contrast-enhanced EUS. Imaging of a pancreatic neuroendocrine tumor after contrast injection. (*Courtesy of* Marc Giovannini, MD, Marseille, France.)

Endoscopic ultrasound scan fine-needle aspiration

The ability of EUS to obtain tissue or core biopsy specimens of pancreatic lesions is one of the most attractive features of endosonography. Before the advent of EUS fine-needle aspiration (EUS-FNA), percutaneous needle aspiration or intraoperative tissue acquisition was needed, but each had its own drawbacks such as malignant needle tract seeding and the invasive morbidity of diagnostic laparoscopy.[52,53] Overall EUS-FNA has a sensitivity of 85% to 94% and specificity of 100% for pancreatic cancer.[54–56] EUS-FNA sensitivity is lower in patients with chronic pancreatitis and a focal mass decreasing to 54% in some reports.[57] Much research has focused on improving the cellular yield of FNA sampling based on needle size selection (FNA needles vary from 19 to 25 gauge), increasing the number of needle passes, "fanning" technique, use of suction, and pull-back methods of removing the stylet. What stands out clearly among these variations of technique is that the availability of on-site cytopathology improves the diagnostic yield of FNA,[58] and when this is unavailable, at least 7 FNA passes are needed to achieve a high sensitivity (83%) for diagnosing malignant pancreatic lesions.[59]

Another variation of EUS tissue sampling technique is the development of fine-needle biopsy, in which core biopsy samples are obtained rather than cellular aspirates from FNA. This technique is particularly suited when there is clinical suspicion for lymphoma or stromal tumors where the tissue architecture needs to be preserved and full examination of the tissue histopathology is essential for accurate diagnosis.[60] Additionally, core biopsy samples allow immunohistochemistry staining and other molecular studies to be performed on the sample. One large, multicentered retrospective cohort study of 109 patients with both intraintestinal and extraintestinal lesions sampled using a 19-gauge fine-needle biopsy device, EchoTip ProCore designed by Cook Endoscopy (Limerick, Ireland) had a technical feasibility rate of 98%, adequate tissue sampling for full histologic evaluation in 89% of cases, and an overall diagnostic accuracy for malignancy of 92.9% with no reported complications.[61]

Pancreatic Cysts

Although the combination of clinical and radiologic data can provide an initial diagnosis in the evaluation of pancreatic cysts, EUS can add additional diagnostic value in indeterminate cysts based on their endosonographic features, cyst fluid analysis for amylase, carcinoembryonic antigen (CEA), and cytology. Generally, all symptomatic or obstructing cysts, even when there is low suspicion for malignancy, should be referred for surgical resection or endoscopic drainage in the case of symptomatic pseudocysts. For asymptomatic pancreatic cysts, initial clinical decision making depends on differentiating between mucinous and nonmucinous cysts because of the malignant potential of mucinous cysts. Pseudocysts on EUS appear as unilocular, anechoic lesions arising within pancreatic parenchyma that has changes consistent with acute or chronic pancreatitis (**Fig. 4**). Fluid aspirate from a pseudocyst has elevated amylase (>5000 U/mL) and lipase (>2000 U/mL) levels.[62] Serous cystadenomas classically have a microcystic or honeycomb appearance with multiple small cysts that together form the lesion and on fluid analysis have a CEA level less than 5 ng/mL (**Fig. 5**). Mucinous cystadenomas are macrocystic, unilocular lesions usually found in the body and tail with viscous, thick mucin on FNA, which may have markedly elevated CEA level on fluid analysis, although a low CEA level does not exclude the possibility of a mucinous lesion. IPMNs are classified as MD-IPMN, which have a mean risk of malignancy of 61%,[63] and side-branch or branch duct IPMN (BD-IPMN), which have much lower rates of malignancy (**Fig. 6**). The International Consensus Guidelines of 2012 for management of IPMN and MCN recommend surgical resection of all MD-IPMN in surgically fit patients to prevent development of malignancy.[63] The management of BD-IPMNs is more controversial. EUS examinations of BD-IPMN should focus on the evaluation of high risk features or predictors of malignancy: solid component or mural nodule, main pancreatic duct dilation ≥ 1 cm, and cyst size ≥ 3 cm^2. The 2015 American Gastroenterological Association guidelines on asymptomatic pancreatic cysts recommend EUS examination only when 2 such high-risk features are present and noninvasive surveillance with MRI in all other cases. Prospective validation of these recommendations is lacking, and clinical practice patterns can vary widely in BD-IPMN surveillance.

Despite the high-resolution imaging provided by EUS, a large multicentered series found that EUS morphology alone had a sensitivity of only 56%, specificity of 45%, and overall accuracy of 51% in distinguishing mucinous and nonmucinous cysts.[64] Furthermore interobserver agreeability is only fair to moderate even among expert sonographers.[65] Retrospective series found EUS with the addition of cytology has a better overall accuracy in differentiating mucinous and nonmucinous cysts of 88%.[66] Newer molecular markers obtained from cyst FNA have also shown some promise in helping differentiate between mucinous and nonmucinous lesions. K-ras

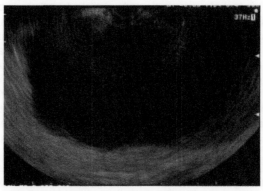

Fig. 4. EUS image of pseudocyst. Anechoic (*black*) cystic lesion with irregular borders, small amount of layering debris inferiorly.

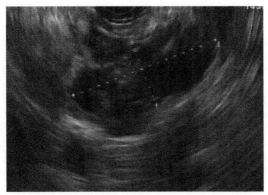

Fig. 5. EUS image of IPMN. A multicystic, irregularly shaped cyst with a possible nodule versus mucin collection is seen by B-mode EUS imaging.

mutations have nearly 100% specificity for mucinous cysts, although sensitivity is lower at 54%.[67] GNAS mutations are also being studied as a specific marker of IPMNs, especially when present in combination with K-ras mutations.[68]

Probe-based confocal laser endomicroscopy

Confocal laser endomicroscopy (CLE) is a novel imaging technology that aims to achieve optical biopsy by providing microscopic-level imaging of the epithelium of the gastrointestinal tract. The examinations are carried out in vivo with real-time image display. In CLE, tissue is illuminated with a low-power laser, and fluorescent light is detected after being reflected from the tissue. CLE relies on tissue fluorescence, and hence a contrast agent, in this case, fluorescein, is used to help distinguish cellular structures that absorb or do not absorb the dye. The probe-based CLE system uses a miniature confocal probe that can be passed through the working channel of a

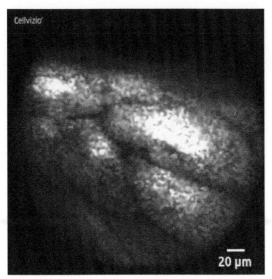

Fig. 6. An nCLE image of IPMN. Papillary projections are seen using AQ Flex probe. (*Courtesy of* Amrita Sethi, Columbia University Medical Center, New York, NY.)

standard endoscope. More recently a needle-based CLE (nCLE) has been developed to access tissue via a 19-gauge EUS-FNA needle to image pancreatic lesions.[69] The procedure is performed with intravenous fluorescein given moments before the examination. The probe is preloaded into the needle and locked at a length that will allow for the tip of the probe to extend just beyond the needle. It is then withdrawn completely into the needle to protect the fragile tip during cyst puncture. Once the needle is properly positioned against the cyst wall or septum, the probe is locked onto the needle pushing the tip beyond the end of the needle and is applied gently to the cyst wall. The nCLE has a field of view of 320 μm and lateral resolution of 3.5 μm. This degree of resolution allows for visualization of structures such as capillary vessels and individual blood cells within, goblet cells, and even polarity of nuclei. In pancreatic cysts, targets for visualization include structures such as microscopic vascular networks or the single ovarian stromal layer that is seen on histologic slides. Other abnormal characteristics that can be seen include dark clumps or hypervascularity, which may be seen in solid lesions such as neuroendocrine tumors (**Fig. 7**). Initial feasibility studies showed the needle probe can be successfully introduced into pancreatic lesions (16 cysts and 2 masses), and high-quality images can be obtained in most of these cases, but notable complications include 2 cases of pancreatitis requiring hospitalization.[69] A follow-up multicentered study of nCLE in pancreatic cysts provided the first description of CLE findings of mucinous cystic neoplasm, where epithelial villous structure was found to have 100% specificity but lower sensitivity of 59% in identifying mucinous cystic neoplasm.[70] The diagnostic yield of nCLE was higher than that of cytology alone and CEA levels for identifying mucinous cystic neoplasms.[70] Use of nCLE in the evaluation of pancreatic cysts remains investigational, and it is associated with an up to 9% complication rate with the most frequent complication being pancreatitis.[69,70] Further large prospective, multicentered trials are needed to validate these early findings and clarify the role of nCLE in pancreatic imaging.

Widespread use of this technology might be hindered by cost, as adoption of CLE requires purchase of a laser unit, processor, and probes. In addition, there is a learning

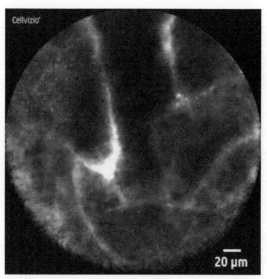

Fig. 7. An nCLE image of neuroendocrine tumor. (*Courtesy of* Amrita Sethi, Columbia University Medical Center, New York, NY.)

curve for the endoscopist that requires supervised training.[71] The procedure itself is not time intensive, especially if the system is prepared in advance. In addition, the needle used for the confocal examination can be used for fluid aspiration and sampling as well. Although a reimbursement code exists for confocal endomicroscopy of the gastrointestinal lumen, the nCLE examination does not have a recognized code.

Chronic Pancreatitis

EUS is well suited to the diagnosis of chronic pancreatitis, as it delineates both pancreatic parenchymal changes and pancreatic ductal changes, which, in early disease, can be missed on cross-sectional imaging. Consensus EUS criteria for chronic pancreatitis were established through the International Working Group in 2007, referred to as the *Rosemont Criteria* (**Box 3**). The criteria were divided into major and minor criteria based on their relative predictive accuracy. A confirmatory diagnosis of chronic pancreatitis was made if there was a combination of 1 major A criteria plus at least 3 minor criteria, 1 major A criteria plus a major B criteria, or 2 major A features.[72] Any other combination of features was considered either suggestive of chronic pancreatitis or indeterminate. If there were less than 2 minor criteria found with no major criteria, then the pancreas was thought to be normal. Since its publication, there remains substantial controversy on the number of criteria needed to meet a definite or even probable diagnosis of chronic pancreatitis, as the Rosemont Classification remains largely a set of expert opinions. Validation of the relative predictive value of each specific criterion and determining the number of criteria needed to optimize the diagnostic accuracy of EUS are ongoing. Furthermore, the interobserver agreement of EUS features for the diagnosis of chronic pancreatitis is relatively poor. Studies of expert endosonographers blinded to clinical information who evaluated videotapes of EUS examinations for chronic pancreatitis

---

Box 3
EUS criteria for diagnosis of chronic pancreatitis (Rosemont criteria)

Major criteria A

Hyperechoic foci that cause shadowing

Major ductal calculi

Major criteria B

Lobularity ($\geq$3 contiguous lobules = honeycombing)

Minor criteria

Cyst (anechoic, round or elliptical with or without septations)

Dilated duct $\geq$3.5 mm in body or >1.5 mm in tail

Irregular duct contour

Dilated side branch

Hyperechoic duct wall

Hyperechoic strands

Hyperechoic foci without shadowing

Lobularity

Data from Catalano MF, Sahai A, Levy M, et al. EUS-based criteria for the diagnosis of chronic pancreatitis: the Rosemont classification. Gastrointest Endosc 2009;69:1251–61.

showed only moderate agreement ($\kappa = 0.45$).[73,74] EUS alone is thus not sufficient for the diagnosis of chronic pancreatitis and must be taken in the context of the clinical presentation, laboratory evaluation, and emerging functional imaging studies such as secretin-enhanced MRI.

EMERGING TECHNOLOGIES

Some experimental work has been done in developing molecular imaging of the pancreas. One method is by combining the technology of confocal endomicroscopy with fluorescence markers to antibodies such as epithelial growth factor receptor or survivin. Both of these proteins are found to be upregulated in pancreatic cancer tissue. In porcine studies, Nakai and colleagues[75] showed the feasibility of using the nCLE probe to visualize areas of uptake of both antihuman epithelial growth factor receptor fluorescein–conjugated monoclonal antibody and antihuman survivin fluorescein–conjugated monoclonal antibody that was previously injected in pancreatic tissue primed with these agents using EUS-guided fine-needle injection. The investigators suggested that this finding showed the ability to perform in vivo functional imaging of pancreatic tissue. Similarly, Konkalmatt and colleagues[76] found that vector-bound Plectin-1 Targeting Peptide (PTP) preferentially targeted pancreatic cancer cells in mouse models that could then be visualized using bioluminescence imaging. These studies offer possibilities that may lead to exciting advances in molecular imaging and understanding pancreatic pathophysiology.[75,76]

SUMMARY

Pancreatic imaging has continued to evolve with the advent of EUS and an increasing interest in real-time, higher-resolution delineation of pancreatic lesions. Newer technology is pushing the future of pancreatic imaging toward optical biopsy, but efforts are also ongoing to improve the diagnostic accuracy of the available tools we have now by refining criteria for assessing, staging, and differentiating the etiology of pancreatic lesions and ensuring greater interobserver reliability in endosonography.

REFERENCES

1. American Cancer Society data as of July 5, 2015. Available at: http://www.cancer.org/cancer/pancreaticcancer/detailedguide/pancreatic-cancer-key-statistics. Accessed July 22, 2015.
2. Vege S, Ziring B, Jain R, et al. American gastroenterological association institute guideline on the diagnosis and management of asymptomatic neoplastic pancreatic cysts. Gastroenterology 2015;148:819–22.
3. Gijón de la Santa L, Pérez Retortillo JA, Camarero Miguel A, et al. Radiology of pancreatic neoplasms: an update. World J Gastrointest Oncol 2014;6(9):330–43.
4. DeWitt J, Devereaux B, Chriswell M, et al. Comparison of endoscopic ultrasound and multidetector computed tomography for detecting and staging pancreatic cancer. Ann Intern Med 2004;141:753–63.
5. Soriano A, Castells A, Ayuso C, et al. Preoperative staging and tumor resectability assessment of pancreatic cancer: prospective study comparing endoscopic ultrasounography, helical computed tomography, magnetic resonance imaging, and angiography. Am J Gastroenterol 2004;99:492–501.
6. Rivadeneira DE, Pochapin M, Grobmyer SR, et al. Comparison of linear array endoscopic ultrasound and helical computed tomography for the staging of periampullary malignancies. Ann Surg Oncol 2003;10:890–7.

7. Ramsay D, Marshall M, Song S, et al. Identification and staging of pancreatic tumours using computed tomography, endoscopic ultrasound and mangafodipir trisodium-enhanced magnetic resonance imaging. Australas Radiol 2004;48: 154–61.
8. Muller MF, Meyenberger C, Bertschinger P, et al. Pancreatic tumors: evaluation with endoscopic US, Ct, and MR imaging. Radiology 1994;190:745–51.
9. Ainsworth AP, Rafaelsen SR, Wamberg PA, et al. Is there a difference in diagnostic accuracy and clinical impact between ednsocopic ultrasounography and magnetic resonance cholangiopancreatography? Endoscopy 2003;35: 1029–32.
10. Fishman EK, Horton KM. Imaging pancreatic cancer: the role of multidetector CT with three dimensional CT angiography. Pancreatology 2001;6:610–24.
11. Brennan DD, Zamboni GA, Raptopoulos VD, et al. Comprehensive preoperative assessment of pancreatic adenocarcinoma with 64-section volumetric CT. Radiographics 2007;27:1653–66.
12. Low G, Panu A, Millo N, et al. Multimodality imaging of neoplastic and nonneoplastic solid lesions of the pancreas. Radiographics 2011;31:993–1015.
13. Freeny PC, Traverso LW, Ryan JA. Diagnosis and staging of pancreatic adenocarcinoma with dynamic computed tomography. Am J Surg 1993;165:600–6.
14. Diehl SJ, Lehmann KJ, Sadick M, et al. Pancreatic cancer: value of dual-phase helical CT in assessing resectability. Radiology 1998;206:373–8.
15. Bluemke DA, Cameron JL, Hruban RH, et al. Potentially resectable pancreatic adenocarcinoma: spiral assessment with surgical and pathologic correlation. Radiology 1995;197:381–5.
16. Tabuchi T, Itoh K, Ohshio G, et al. Tumor staging of pancreatic adenocarcinoma using early and late-phase helical CT. AJR Am J Roentgenol 1999;173:375–80.
17. Ichikawa T, Hardome H, Hachiya J, et al. Pancreatic ductal adenocarcinoma: a preoperative assessment with helical CT versus dynamic MR imaging. Radiology 1997;202:655–62.
18. Wang Y, Miller FH, Chen ZE, et al. Diffusionweighted MR imaging of solid and cystic lesions of the pancreas. Radiographics 2011;31:E47–64.
19. Kartalis N, Lindholm TL, Aspelin P, et al. Diffusion-weighted magnetic resonance imaging of pancreas tumors. Eur Radiol 2009;19:1981–90.
20. Taylor AC, Little AF, Hennessy OF, et al. Prospective assessment of magnetic resonance cholangiopancreatography for noninvasive imaging of the biliary tree. Gastrointest Endosc 2002;55:17–22.
21. Hekimoglu K, Ustundag Y, Dusak A, et al. MRCP vs. ERCP in the evaluation of biliary pathologies: review of current literature. J Dig Dis 2008;9:162–9.
22. Reddy RP, Smyrk TC, Zapiach M, et al. Pancreatic mucinous cystic neoplasm defined by ovarian stroma: demographics, clinical features, and prevalence of cancer. Clin Gastroenterol Hepatol 2004;2:1026–31.
23. Campbell F, Azadeh B. Cystic neoplasms of the exocrine pancreas. Histopathology 2008;52:539–51.
24. Zamboni G, Scarpa A, Bogina G, et al. Mucinous cystic tumors of the pancreas: clinicopathological features, prognosis, and relationship to other mucinous cystic tumors. Am J Surg Pathol 1999;23:410–22.
25. Crippa S, Salvia R, Warshaw AL, et al. Mucinous cystic neoplasm of the pancreas is not an aggressive entity: lessons from 163 resected patients. Ann Surg 2008; 247:571–9.
26. Sugiyama M, Izumisato Y, Abe N, et al. Predictive factors for malignancy in intraductal papillarymucinous tumours of the pancreas. Br J Surg 2003;90:1244–9.

27. Salvia R, Fernández-del Castillo C, Bassi C, et al. Main-duct intraductal papillary mucinous neoplasms of the pancreas: clinical predictors of malignancy and long-term survival following resection. Ann Surg 2004;239:678–85.
28. Schmidt CM, White PB, Waters JA, et al. Intraductal papillary mucinous neoplasms: predictors of malignant and invasive pathology. Ann Surg 2007;246:644–51.
29. Balci NC, Semelka RC. Radiologic features of cystic, endocrine and other pancreatic neoplasms. Eur J Radiol 2001;38:113–9.
30. Irie H, Honda H, Aibe H, et al. MR cholangiopancreatographic differentiation of benign and malignant intraductal mucin-producing tumors of the pancreas. AJR Am J Roentgenol 2000;174:1403–8.
31. Berland LL, Silverman SG, Gore RM, et al. Managing incidental findings on abdominal CT: white paper of the ACR incidental findings committee. J Am Coll Radiol 2010;7:754–73.
32. Sainani NI, Saokar A, Deshpande V, et al. Comparative performance of MDCT and MRI with MR cholangiopancreatography in characterizing small pancreatic cysts. AJR Am J Roentgenol 2009;193:722–73.
33. Kim YC, Choi JY, Chung YE, et al. Comparison of MRI and endoscopic ultrasound in the characterization of pancreatic cystic lesions. AJR Am J Roentgenol 2010; 195:947–52.
34. Hunt GC, Faigel DO. Assessment of EUS for diagnosing, staging, and determining resectability of pancreatic cancer: a review. Gastrointest Endosc 2002;55:232–7.
35. Gress F, Hawes RH, Savides TJ, et al. Role of EUS in the preoperative staging of pancreatic cancer: a large single-center experience. Gastrointest Endosc 1999; 50:786–91.
36. Palazzo L, Roseau G, Gayet B, et al. Endoscopic ultrasonography in the diagnosis and staging of pancreatic adenocarcinoma. Endoscopy 1993;25:143–50.
37. Agarwal B, Abu-Hamda E, Molke KL, et al. Endoscopic ultrasound-guided fine needle aspiration and multidetector spiral CT in the diagnosis of pancreatic pancreatic cancer. Am J Gastroenterol 2004;99:844–50.
38. Legmann P, Vignaux O, Dousset B, et al. Pancreatic tumors: comparison of dual-phase helical CT and endoscopic sonography. AJR Am J Roentgenol 1998;170: 1315–22.
39. Nakaizumi A, Uehara H, Ilishi H, et al. Endoscopic ultrasonography in diagnosis and staging of pancreatic cancer. Dig Dis Sci 1995;40:696–700.
40. Tierney WM, Francis IR, Eckhauser F, et al. The accuracy of EUS and helical CT in the assessment of vascular invasion by peripapillary malignancy. Gastrointest Endosc 2001;53:182–8.
41. Rosch T, Dittler HJ, Seigel J, et al. Endoscopic ultrasound criteria for vascular invasion in the staging of cancer of the head of the pancreas: a blind reevaluation of videotapes. Gastrointest Endosc 2000;52:469–77.
42. Ngamruengphong S, Feng Li, Ying Zhou, et al. EUS and survival in patients with pancreatic cacner in a population-based study. Gastrointest Endosc 2010;72: 78–83.
43. Al-haddad M, Dewitt J. EUS in pancreatic tumors. In: Hawes R, Fockens P, editors. Endosonography. Philadelphia: Elsevier; 2011. p. 148–65.
44. Janssen J, Schlörer E, Greiner L. EUS elastography of the pancreas: feasibility and pattern description of the normal pancreas, chronic pancreatitis, and focal pancreatic lesions. Gastrointest Endosc 2007;65:971–8.
45. Giovannini M, Hookey LC, Bories E, et al. Endoscopic ultrasound elastography: the first step towards virtual biopsy? Preliminary results in 49 patients. Endoscopy 2006;38:344–8.

46. Hirche TO, Ignee A, Barreiros AT, et al. Indications and limitations of endoscopic ultrasound elastography for evaluation of focal pancreatic lesions. Endoscopy 2008;40:910–7.
47. Săftoiu A, Vilmann P, Gorunescu F, et al. Accuracy of endoscopic ultrasound elastography used for differential diagnosis of focal pancreatic masses: a multicenter study. Endoscopy 2011;43:596–603.
48. Soares JB, Iglesias-Garcia J, Gonacalves B, et al. INterobserver agreement of EUS elastography in the evaluation of solid pancreatic lesions. Endosc Ultrasound 2015;4(3):244–9.
49. Morin SH, Lim AK, Cobbold JF, et al. Use of second generation contrast-enhanced ultrasound in the assessment of focal liver lesions. World J Gastroenterol 2007;13:5963–70.
50. Teshima CW, Sandha G. Endoscopic ultrasound in the diagnosis and treatment of pancreatic disease. World J Gastroenterol 2014;29:9976–89.
51. Gong TT, Hu DM, Zhu Q. Contrast-enhanced EUS for differential diagnosis of pancreatic mass lesions: a meta-analysis. Gastrointest Endosc 2012;76:301–9.
52. Smith EP, Marcdonald JS, Schein PS, et al. Cutaneous seeding of pancreatic cancer by skinny needle aspiration biopsy. Arch Intern Med 1980;140:855.
53. Ferrcucci IT, Wittenberg J, Margolies MN, et al. Malignant seeding of the tract after thin-needle aspiration biopsy. Radiology 1979;130:345–6.
54. Cahn M, Chang K, Nguyen P, et al. Impact of endoscopic ultrasound with fine-needle aspiration on the surgical management of pancreatic cancer. Am J Surg 1996;172:470–2.
55. Varadarajulu S, Tamhane A, Eloubeidi MA. Yield of EUS-guided FNA of pancreatic masses in the presence or the absence of chronic pancreatitis. Gastrointest Endosc 2005;62:728–36.
56. Gress F, Gottlieb K, Sherman S, et al. Endoscopic ultrasound-guided fine-needle aspiration biopsy using linear array and radial scanning endosonography. Gastrointest Endosc 1997;45:243–50.
57. Fritscher-Ravens A, Brand L, Knofel WT, et al. Comparison of endoscopic ultrasound-guided fine needle aspiration for focal pancreatic lesions in patients with normal parenchyma and chronic pancreatitis. Am J Gastroenterol 2002;97:2768–75.
58. Iglesias-Garcia J, Dominguez-Munoz JE, Abdulkader I, et al. Influence of on-site cytopathology evaluation on the diagnostic accuracy of endoscopic ultrasound-guided fine needle aspiration (EUS-FNA) of solid pancreatic masses. Am J Gastroenterol 2011;106:1705–10.
59. LeBlanc JK, Ciaccia D, Al-Assi MT, et al. Optimal number of EUS-guided fine needle passes needed to obtain a correct diagnosis. Gastrointest Endosc 2004;59:475–81.
60. Mesa H, Stelow EB, Stanley MW, et al. Diagnosis of non-primary pancreatic neoplasms by endoscopic ultrasound-guided fine-needle aspiration. Diagn Cytopathol 2004;31:313–8.
61. Iglesias-Garcia J, Poley JW, Larghi A, et al. Feasibility and yield of a new EUS histology needle: results from a multicenter, pooled, cohort study. Gastrointest Endosc 2011;73:1189–96.
62. Penman I, Lennon AM. EUS in the evaluation of pancreatic cysts. In: Hawes R, Fockens P, editors. Endosonography. Philadelphia: Elsevier; 2011. p. 166–77.
63. Tanaka M, Fernandez-del Castillo C, Adsay V, et al. International consensus guidelines 2012 for the management of IPMN and MCN of the pancreas. Pancreatology 2012;12:183–97.

64. Brugge WR, Lewandrowski K, Lee-Lewandrowski E, et al. Diagnosis of pancreatic cystic neoplasms: a report of the cooperative pancreatic cyst study. Gastroenterology 2004;126:1330–6.
65. de Jong K, Verlaan T, Dijkgraaf MG, et al. Interobserver agreement for endosonography in the diagnosis of pancreatic cysts. Endoscopy 2011;43:579–84.
66. Chebib I, Yaeger K, Mino-Kenudson M, et al. The role of cytopathology and cyst fluid analysis in the preoperative diagnosis and management of pancreatic cysts >3 cm. Cancer Cytopathol 2014;122:804–9.
67. Nikiforova MN, Khalid A, Fasanella KE, et al. Integration of KRAS testing in the diagnosis of pancreatic cystic lesions: a clinical experience of 618 pancreatic cysts. Mod Pathol 2013;26:1478–87.
68. Singhi AD, Nikiforova MN, Fasanella KE, et al. Preoperative GNAS and KRAS testing in the diagnosis of pancreatic mucinous cysts. Clin Cancer Res 2014; 20:4381–9.
69. Konda V, Aslanian HR, Wallace M, et al. First assessment of needle-based confocal laser endomicroscopy during EUS-FNA procedures of the pancreas. Gastrointest Endosc 2011;74(5):1049–60.
70. Konda V, Meining A, Laith HJ, et al. A pilot study of in vivo identification of pancreatic cystic neoplasms with needle-based confocal laser endomicroscopy under endosonographic guidance. Endoscopy 2013;45(12):1006–13.
71. Talreja JP, Sethi A, Jamidar PA, et al. Interpretation of probe-based confocal laser endomicroscopy of indeterminate biliary strictures: is there any interobserver agreement? Dig Dis Sci 2012;57(12):3299–302.
72. Catalano MF, Sahai A, Levy M, et al. EUS-based criteria for the diagnosis of chronic pancreatitis: the Rosemont classification. Gastrointest Endosc 2009;69: 1251–61.
73. Wallace MB, Hawes RH, Durkalski V, et al. The reliability of EUS for the diagnosis of chronic pancreatitis: interobserver agreement among experienced endosonographers. Gastrointest Endosc 2001;53:294–9.
74. Topazian M, Enders F, Kimmey M, et al. Interobserver agreement for EUS findings in familial pancreatic-cancer kindreds. Gastrointest Endosc 2007;66:62–7.
75. Nakai Y, Shinoura S, Ahluwalia A. In vivo visualization of epidermal growth factor receptor and surviving expression in porcine pancreas using endoscopic ultrasound guided fine needle imaging with confocal laser-induced endomicroscopy. J Physiol Pharmacol 2012;63(6):577–80.
76. Konkalmatt PR, Deng D, Thomas S. Plectin-1 targeted AAV vector for the molecular imaging of pancreatic cancer. Front Oncol 2013;3:1–6.

Screening for Pancreatic Cancer in High-risk Populations

Shilpa Grover, MD, MPH*, Kunal Jajoo, MD

KEYWORDS

- Pancreatic cancer • Hereditary • Screening • Peutz-Jeghers • BRCA
- Lynch syndrome • IPMN • PanIN

KEY POINTS

- Approximately 10% of pancreatic cancer cases are estimated to have an underlying hereditary basis. Of these, only 20% are caused by a known genetic syndrome. Most are caused by nonsyndromic aggregation of pancreatic cancer cases or familial pancreatic cancer.
- Assessment of family cancer history is essential to identify individuals who may benefit from genetic evaluation, testing for underlying cancer susceptibility genes, and screening for pancreatic cancer.
- Screening aims to identify preinvasive lesions with high-grade neoplastic changes that are significantly associated with an increased risk for invasive pancreatic cancer (pancreatic intraepithelial neoplasia-3 and intraductal papillary mucinous neoplasm with high-grade dysplasia).
- Endoscopic ultrasonography and MRI/magnetic resonance cholangiopancreatography can detect pancreatic cancer precursor lesions in high-risk individuals but have limitations.
- Novel biomarkers have the potential to inform the diagnosis and management of pancreatic cancer precursor lesions detected on imaging.

INTRODUCTION

Pancreatic adenocarcinoma is the fourth leading cause of cancer-related death in the United States and the eighth leading cause worldwide.[1] Surgical resection is the only potentially curative treatment of exocrine pancreatic cancer. However, because of the late presentation at diagnosis, only 15% to 20% of patients are candidates for surgery.

Division of Gastroenterology, Brigham and Women's Hospital, Harvard Medical School, 75 Francis Street, Boston, MA 02115, USA
* Corresponding author.
E-mail address: Shilpa.Grover@bwh.harvard.edu

Gastroenterol Clin N Am 45 (2016) 117–127
http://dx.doi.org/10.1016/j.gtc.2015.10.001

Early detection of pancreatic cancer with curative resection can improve survival.[2,3] Population-based screening for pancreatic cancer is not cost-effective given the low incidence of pancreatic cancer and the low positive predictive value of current screening modalities. However, individuals at increased risk for pancreatic cancer may benefit from screening to detect early pancreatic neoplasia and screening may be cost-effective.[4,5]

EPIDEMIOLOGY

Approximately 10% of pancreatic cancer cases are estimated to have an underlying hereditary basis.[6] Of these, only 20% are caused by a known genetic syndrome (**Table 1**).[7]

Familial Pancreatic Cancer

Familial pancreatic cancer (FPC) has been defined by consensus opinion as affecting families with at least 2 first-degree relatives (FDRs) with pancreatic cancer without a known pancreatic cancer–associated hereditary syndrome.

The risk of pancreatic cancer in FPC families increases with the number of affected FDRs. Other important determinants of pancreatic cancer risk in FPC families include the age at pancreatic cancer diagnosis, the family size, and the number of first-degree relatives with pancreatic cancer in the family. Genetic anticipation has been noted in 65% to 80% of individuals from FPC families.[8] In one prospective study that included 838 FPC kindreds, individuals with 1 affected FDR had a 4.5-fold increased risk compared with the general population.[9] Those with 2 and 3 or more affected FDRs with pancreatic cancer had a 6.4-fold and 32-fold increased risk of developing pancreatic cancer, respectively.

Table 1
Syndromes associated with increased risk of pancreatic cancer

Syndrome	Gene	Estimated Lifetime Risk of Pancreatic Cancer (%)
Peutz-Jeghers syndrome	STK11	11–36
FAMMM	p16/CDKN2A	10–17
Hereditary breast and ovarian cancer	BRCA2 BRCA1	5 3.6
Fanconi anemia, breast cancer	PALB2	Unknown
Lynch syndrome	MLH1, MSH2, MSH6, PMS2, EPCAM	3.7
Li-Fraumeni syndrome	p53	Unknown
Familial adenomatous polyposis	APC	2
Ataxia-telangiectasia	ATM	Unknown
Hereditary pancreatitis	PRSS1	40
Familial pancreatic cancer 1 FDR 2 FDR ≥3 FDR	Majority unknown	6 8–12 40

Abbreviations: FAMMM, familial atypical multiple mole and melanoma; FDR, first-degree relative.

Segregation models suggest that pancreatic cancer in FPC families may be caused by an autosomal dominant susceptibility gene with reduced penetrance, carried by approximately 7 per 1000 individuals.[10] Initial studies also suggested that germline *BRCA2* mutations may be found in 15% to 17% of FPC kindreds with an incident pancreatic cancer.[11–13] However, in larger cohort studies, deleterious *BRCA2* mutations were detected in only 6% of moderate-risk and high-risk families.[14] Mutations in the partner and localizer of the *BRCA2* (*PALB2*) gene and ataxia-telangiectasia mutated (*ATM*) gene have also been identified in FPC kindreds.[15] However, the underlying susceptibility gene that explains most cases of pancreatic cancer caused by an inherited predisposition have not been identified.

The complexity in pancreatic cancer risk assessment has been the impetus for the development of a prediction model. The PancPRO model takes into account an individual's age, personal and family history of cancer, age at cancer diagnosis, and family size, and can provide a quantitative estimate of the absolute lifetime pancreatic cancer risk without knowing the gene responsible for the aggregation of pancreatic cancer in a family.[16]

Pancreatic Cancer Associated with Inherited Cancer Syndromes

Peutz-Jeghers syndrome

Peutz-Jeghers syndrome (PJS) is an autosomal dominant hamartomatous polyposis syndrome with high penetrance caused by a mutation in the *STK11* gene. PJS is characterized by multiple hamartomatous polyps and mucocutaneous pigmentation. Hamartomatous polyps can develop throughout the gastrointestinal tract but most commonly occur in the small bowel. Gastrointestinal polyps usually develop in the first decade of life and most patients are symptomatic by the age of 30 years. Hamartomatous polyps can also occur in the urinary bladder, renal pelvis, nasopharynx, and lungs. More than 95% of individuals with PJS have mucocutaneous pigmentation that develops early in life and then fades after puberty, with the exception of lesions on the buccal mucosa.

Individuals with PJS have an estimated lifetime risk of pancreatic cancer of 11% to 36%, with a mean age of 41 years at pancreatic cancer diagnosis.[6,17] PJS is also associated with an increased risk for colorectal, gastric, and small bowel cancers, with lifetime risks of 39%, 29%, and 13%, respectively. In addition, individuals with PJS are at an increased risk for cancers of the breast, ovary, cervix, uterus, testicle, and lung. A clinical diagnosis of PJS requires the presence of any one of the following: 2 or more histologically confirmed Peutz-Jeghers (PJ) polyps; any number of PJ polyps in an individual who has a family history of PJS in a close relative; characteristic mucocutaneous pigmentation in an individual who has a family history of PJS in a close relative; or any number of PJ polyps in an individual who also has characteristic mucocutaneous pigmentation. Genetic testing for mutation in the *STK11* gene in an individual who meets clinical criteria for PJS serves to establish the diagnosis of PJS.

Familial atypical multiple mole and melanoma

Familial atypical multiple mole and melanoma (FAMMM) is an autosomal dominantly inherited syndrome caused by mutations in the *CDKN2A* gene. The *CDKN2A* gene encodes the p16 protein, which functions as a cell cycle regulator. FAMMM is characterized by multiple melanocytic nevi, atypical melanocytic nevi, and an increased risk for early onset melanoma. Individuals with a clinical diagnosis of FAMMM have a 13-fold to 22-fold increased risk of pancreatic cancer compared with the general population.[18] In individuals with the Leiden founder mutation in the *CDKN2A* gene, the risk of pancreatic cancer is increased 47-fold.[19] Individuals with FAMMM are also at an increased risk for cancer of the respiratory tract, eye/brain, oropharynx, and nonmelanoma skin cancer.

Hereditary breast cancer

Hereditary breast and ovarian cancer syndrome is characterized by early onset breast and/or ovarian cancer caused by autosomal dominant, highly penetrant, germline mutations in BRCA1 and BRCA2. Individuals with germline mutations in BRCA2 have a 3.5-fold to 5.9-fold increased risk of developing pancreatic cancer, with a mean age of 63 years at diagnosis.[11,20,21] Germline BRCA2 mutations account for the highest proportion of known causes of inherited pancreatic cancer. BRCA2 mutations have been found in 6% to 17% of tested FPC kindreds with an incident pancreatic cancer.[11,12,14] It is estimated that 1.7% to 10% of patients of Ashkenazi Jewish ancestry with pancreatic cancer carry a BRCA mutation and most these patients lack a family history of BRCA-associated cancers.[22,23]

Individuals with germline mutations in BRCA1 have a lower risk of pancreatic adenocarcinoma compared with those with a BRCA2 mutation.[24] In one cohort study that included 11,847 individuals from 699 families segregating a BRCA1 mutation, the risk of pancreatic cancer was increased 2-fold compared with the general population. However, patients were ascertained for young age of onset of breast and/or ovarian cancers and estimates of cancer risk may be lower in FPC families ascertained through pancreatic cancer probands.

Approximately 1% of hereditary breast cancers are caused by germline mutations in the PALB2 gene. The PALB2 protein binds with the BRCA2 protein and stabilizes key nuclear structures needed for DNA repair.[25] Mutations in the PALB2 gene confer an increased risk of both breast and pancreatic cancer and have been identified in 2% to 5% of FPC families.[26,27] Although the absolute risk for pancreatic cancer in individuals with a PALB2 mutation is unknown, given the similarities in gene function of PALB2 and the BRCA genes, the risk of pancreatic cancer is likely to be comparable.[28]

Lynch syndrome

Lynch syndrome or hereditary nonpolyposis colorectal cancer is caused by germline mutations in mismatch repair genes MLH1, MSH2, MSH6, or PMS2, or deletions in the EPCAM gene that result in downstream promotor hypermethylation and silencing of MSH2. Lynch syndrome is the most common inherited familial colorectal cancer syndrome and is characterized by early onset colorectal cancer with a lifetime risk of 60% to 80%. Individuals with Lynch syndrome are at an increased risk for cancers of the endometrium, ovary, stomach, small bowel, urinary tract, and brain.[29] The risk of pancreatic cancer in individuals with Lynch syndrome is increased 9-fold to 11-fold compared with the general population.[30,31] Pancreatic adenocarcinomas in patients with Lynch syndrome characteristically show medullary histology with microsatellite instability and loss of expression of mismatch repair proteins.[32] In one study that evaluated 47 pancreatic cancer cases from 31 families with Lynch syndrome, the cumulative risk of pancreatic cancer in individuals with Lynch syndrome was 1.3% by age 50 years and 3.7% by age 70 years.[30]

Li-Fraumeni syndrome

Li-Fraumeni syndrome (LFS) is an inherited autosomal dominant disorder caused by a germline mutation in the tp53 tumor suppressor gene. LFS is characterized by early onset breast cancer, sarcomas, adrenocortical carcinoma, and brain tumors.[33,34] Individuals with a tp53 mutation also have a 7-fold increased risk of pancreatic cancer compared with the general population.

Familial adenomatous polyposis

Familial adenomatous polyposis (FAP) is an autosomal dominant disorder caused by mutations in the *APC* gene, which encodes a protein that functions as a tumor suppressor and regulates the Wnt pathway. In the classic form of FAP, patients have hundreds or thousands of adenomatous polyps that typically develop during adolescence. A milder, attenuated form of FAP is characterized by fewer than 100 adenomas that are diagnosed at a later age (mean age of 44 years). In the absence of intervention, individuals with FAP have a nearly 100% risk of developing colorectal cancer in their lifetime. They are also at increased risk of extracolonic cancers, including duodenal and thyroid cancer, childhood hepatoblastoma, and central nervous system tumors. There are limited data with regard to the risk of pancreatic cancer in individuals with FAP. However, in one study, individuals with FAP had a 4.5-fold increased risk for pancreatic adenocarcinoma compared with the general population with an absolute lifetime risk of approximately 2%.[35,36]

Ataxia-telangiectasia

Ataxia-telangiectasia is caused by biallelic deleterious mutations in the *ATM* gene. The ATM protein is a serine/threonine kinase involved in DNA repair. Ataxia-telangiectasia is characterized by ataxia, oculocutaneous telangiectasias, radiation sensitivity, immune deficiency, and an increased incidence of malignancy. Monoallelic mutations in the *ATM* gene are associated with a 3-fold increased risk of pancreatic cancer and are found in 2.4% of FPC families.[15,37]

Hereditary pancreatitis

Hereditary pancreatitis is characterized by chronic pancreatitis caused by recurrent attacks of acute pancreatitis. Hereditary pancreatitis is associated with mutations in the *PRSS1* gene, which encodes cationic trypsinogen. The 2 most common mutations in *PRSS1*, R122H and N29I, have a high penetrance.[38]

Normally, cationic trypsinogen is secreted by the pancreas into the duodenum where it is ultimately cleaved into trypsin, which in turn aids proteolysis. Mutations in *PRSS1* result in premature activation of trypsinogen resulting in pancreatic inflammation and pancreatitis. Most affected individuals develop symptoms before age 20 years and often before the age of 5 years. Individuals with hereditary pancreatitis have a 53-fold increased risk of pancreatic cancer compared with the general population. The estimated lifetime risk of pancreatic cancer in individuals with hereditary pancreatitis is 40%, with an average age of 57 years at pancreatic cancer diagnosis.[39]

GENETIC EVALUATION IN INDIVIDUALS AT RISK FOR HEREDITARY PANCREATIC CANCER

Genetic evaluation should be considered for individuals with pancreatic ductal adenocarcinoma whose personal and/or family histories of cancer are concerning for a hereditary cancer predisposition. Features that are suggestive of an inherited predisposition include the presence of multiple family members with the same or associated cancers, early age of onset of polyps or cancer (before age 50 years), multiple primary malignancies, cancers in multiple generations of a family, rare tumors (eg, male breast cancer), unusual histology (eg, medullary carcinoma of the pancreas), and cancers in geographic or ethnic populations known to be associated with a high carrier frequency (eg, Ashkenazi Jewish). Genetic evaluation in patients with suspected FPC should include analysis of mutations in *BRCA1/2*, *CDKN2A*, *PALB2*, and *ATM* genes.[33] In addition, genetic evaluation for PJS, Lynch syndrome, and hereditary pancreatitis should also be considered if an individual's personal and/or family history meet criteria for these syndromes.

MANAGEMENT OF INDIVIDUALS AT RISK FOR PANCREATIC CANCER
Prevention Strategies to Reduce Cancer Risk

Patients should be counseled against smoking, which is a known risk factor for pancreatic cancer that further increases the risk in families with FPC. In one nested case-control study that included 251 members of 28 FPC families, smoking was an independent risk factor for pancreatic cancer (odds ratio [OR], 3.7; 95% confidence interval, 1.8 to 7.6). Smokers developed pancreatic cancer a decade earlier compared with nonsmokers (59 vs 69 years of age).[40] The risk of pancreatic cancer was greatest in men and in individuals younger than 50 years (OR, 5.2 and 7.6, respectively). In addition, individuals with hereditary pancreatitis should be advised to consume a low-fat diet.[41]

Screening for Early Detection of Pancreatic Cancer

Precursors of pancreatic adenocarcinoma

Intraductal papillary mucinous neoplasm (IPMN) and pancreatic intraepithelial neoplasia (PanIN) are well-characterized lesions that give rise to pancreatic adenocarcinoma. IPMN is a grossly visible mucin-producing epithelial neoplasm that can involve the main pancreatic duct, branch ducts, or both. Lesions involving the main pancreatic duct and those with mural nodules carry a higher risk of progression to adenocarcinoma. PanIN is a microscopic noninvasive neoplasm involving small ducts of the pancreas formed by metaplasia and proliferation of ductal epithelium. PanIN lesions show varying degrees of dysplasia that can range in severity from mild to severe (PanIN-1 to PanIN-3).[42] However, the rate of progression of PanIN lesions to adenocarcinoma is unclear.

Outcomes of screening

Screening aims to identify preinvasive lesions with high-grade neoplastic changes that are significantly associated with increased risk for invasive pancreatic cancer (PanIN-3 and IPMN with high-grade dysplasia).

Both the prevalence of IPMN and PanIN lesions and their grade are higher in patients with FPC compared with controls.[43] High-grade precursor lesions in the pancreas of individuals with FPC are often multifocal.[44] Imaging in high-risk families can detect precancerous changes in the pancreas but the reported diagnostic yield has varied widely based on the study methods, screening modality used, and the age at baseline screening. In a large prospective study of 216 high-risk individuals who underwent screening with computed tomography (CT), MRI, and endoscopic ultrasonography (EUS), 92 (42%) had at least 1 pancreatic mass, and 85 were reported to have either proven or suspected neoplasms (82 IPMN and 3 neuroendocrine tumors).[45] However, only 5 individuals underwent surgical resection of the pancreas, of whom 3 (1.4%) were found to have high-grade pancreatic dysplasia in less than 3-cm IPMNs and multiple intraepithelial neoplasias.

Screening for pancreatic cancer has several limitations. High-grade microscopic PanIN may not be detected by imaging. In one study that included 5 of 125 individuals at risk for FPC who underwent surgery for indeterminate branch duct IPMN on MRI, the location of the most dysplastic histologic lesions (PanIN-3) in the pancreas did not correspond with the preoperatively detected lesions and they were not visible on preoperative imaging.[46] It is also unclear whether screening for pancreatic cancer in high-risk individuals improves survival. Screening for pancreatic cancer is associated with the risk of misdiagnosis and treatment of low-risk pancreatic lesions that would not have affected morbidity or mortality during the patient's lifetime.

Screening Modalities

Imaging

Magnetic resonance cholangiopancreatography (MRCP) and EUS are the two main imaging modalities for screening for pancreatic cancer. Secretin-enhanced MRCP further improves sensitivity of MRCP for detecting smaller ductal lesions.[47] MRI/MRCP can visualize other intra-abdominal organs and also has the advantage of avoiding the radiation exposure but is limited by its cost and availability.

EUS can accurately detect IPMNs and visualize mural nodules.[48] Multifocal PanINs with foci of lobulocentric atrophy produce a mosaic of fibrosis, atrophy, and uninvolved parenchyma that resemble changes of chronic pancreatitis.[44] EUS findings including heterogeneous parenchyma, hypoechoic nodules, hyperechoic main-duct walls, and discrete masses have a high positive predictive value for PanIN in high-risk individuals.[49] Targeted imaging agents, such as those that detect plectin, a cell-surface protein expressed in PanIN-3 lesions, may further improve the detection of noncystic pancreatic lesions.[50] However, EUS is limited by significant interobserver variability in interpretation of findings, cost, and the risks associated with endoscopy.[51]

CT and endoscopic retrograde cholangiopancreatography (ERCP) have also been used to screen for pancreatic cancer in high-risk individuals. CT is a rapid, high-resolution imaging modality that can visualize the pancreas and other abdominal/pelvic organs. However, CT has a low sensitivity for small lesions in high-risk populations.[45] CT also has the disadvantage of exposure to radiation, which becomes particularly important to consider when repeated screening is required. ERCP is not recommended for screening because studies have shown that it does not improve the diagnostic yield and is associated with the risk of pancreatitis.[52]

Few studies have compared these imaging modalities directly. In a prospective study in which 216 individuals at increased risk of pancreatic cancer underwent CT, MRI/MRCP, and EUS, screening with MRI/MRCP and EUS had a significantly higher sensitivity in detecting cystic or solid lesions compared with CT scan (77%, 79%, and 14%, respectively).[45] MRI, EUS, and CT detected subcentimeter cysts in 33%, 36%, and 11% of patients, respectively. The concordance between EUS and MRI/MRCP for detection of any pancreatic lesion was significantly higher compared with EUS and CT scan (91% vs 73%).

Biomarkers

Limitations of current screening modalities in identifying microscopic dysplasia and characterizing small cysts have led to the evaluation of biomarkers in pancreatic fluid. Somatic mutations in *GNAS* have been identified in 66% of IPMN lesions and are not found in other types of cystic neoplasms of the pancreas or in invasive adenocarcinomas not associated with IPMN.[53] In a study that included 291 subjects with a familial predisposition to pancreatic cancer who underwent pancreatic screening and controls (normal pancreas, chronic pancreatitis, sporadic IPMN, or other neoplasms), secretin-stimulated pancreatic fluid samples were evaluated for somatic *GNAS* mutations.[54] *GNAS* mutations were detected in the pancreatic fluid of 50 of 78 familial and sporadic IPMN (64%), 15 of 33 (46%) individuals with only diminutive cysts, but none of the 57 disease controls. In addition, mutant *GNAS* detected in baseline fluid samples was associated with the emergence of a new cyst at follow-up.

The *tp53* gene is mutated in approximately 70% of invasive pancreatic cancers and mutations occur late in the progression of PanIN lesions.[55,56] In a study in which 180 individuals at high risk for pancreatic cancer underwent *tp53* mutational analysis of secretin-stimulated pancreatic fluid, *tp53* mutations were detected only in patients with PanIN and IPMN with intermediate-grade (15%) and high-grade dysplasia (43%) and pancreatic ductal adenocarcinoma (67%).[57] Mutations in *tp53* were not detected in any low-grade IPMN or PanIN-1 lesions. Additional studies are needed to validate these results and define the role of mutant *tp53* and *GNAS* in the evaluation of patients at high risk for pancreatic cancer.

Recommendations for pancreatic cancer screening
Current guidelines are primarily based on evidence of increased risk, rather than a proven efficacy of screening for pancreatic cancer in high-risk individuals.[28,33] Screening for pancreatic cancer is recommended in mutation carriers of hereditary syndromes associated with increased risk of pancreatic cancer (Peutz-Jeghers, hereditary pancreatitis, FAMMM) or members of FPC kindreds with an FDR affected with pancreatic cancer.[33] In *BRCA1/BRCA2*, *PALB2*, *ATM*, and Lynch syndrome families, surveillance should be limited to mutation carriers with a first- or second-degree relative affected with pancreatic cancer.

Screening should be performed annually with EUS and/or MRI/MRCP starting at age 50 years, or 10 years younger than the earliest age of pancreatic cancer in the family.[28,33] It is our practice to alternate screening with EUS and MRI/MRCP. In individuals with PJS, screening for pancreatic cancer should begin at age 35 years. Given the limitation in screening and the complexity in management of suspected lesions, patients should be screened and managed by a multidisciplinary team at high-volume centers in the setting of an active research protocol.

SUMMARY

Individuals with FPC and those with inherited syndromes associated with an increased risk of pancreatic cancer may benefit from screening for pancreatic cancer. Current guidelines recommend imaging with EUS and MRI/MRCP in high-risk individuals in order to identify pancreatic cancer precursor lesions. Imaging has a significant yield in appropriately selected, high-risk individuals, but it has limitations. The use of biomarkers as an adjunct to imaging has the potential to inform the diagnosis and management of lesions detected during the course of screening. However, studies are needed to determine whether treating premalignant lesions detected on imaging in high-risk individuals is associated with an improvement in survival.

REFERENCES

1. Siegel R, Ma J, Zou Z, et al. Cancer statistics, 2014. CA Cancer J Clin 2014;64:9.
2. Yeo CJ, Cameron JL. Prognostic factors in ductal pancreatic cancer. Langenbecks Arch Surg 1998;383:129.
3. Shimizu Y, Yasui K, Matsueda K, et al. Small carcinoma of the pancreas is curable: new computed tomography finding, pathological study and postoperative results from a single institute. J Gastroenterol Hepatol 2005;20:1591.
4. Rulyak SJ, Kimmey MB, Veenstra DL, et al. Cost-effectiveness of pancreatic cancer screening in familial pancreatic cancer kindreds. Gastrointest Endosc 2003;57:23.
5. Pandharipande PV, Heberle C, Dowling EC, et al. Targeted screening of individuals at high risk for pancreatic cancer: results of a simulation model. Radiology 2015;275:177.
6. Resta N, Pierannunzio D, Lenato GM, et al. Cancer risk associated with STK11/LKB1 germline mutations in Peutz-Jeghers syndrome patients: results of an Italian multicenter study. Dig Liver Dis 2013;45:606.

7. Hruban RH, Canto MI, Goggins M, et al. Update on familial pancreatic cancer. Adv Surg 2010;44:293.

8. McFaul CD, Greenhalf W, Earl J, et al. Anticipation in familial pancreatic cancer. Gut 2006;55:252.

9. Klein AP, Brune KA, Petersen GM, et al. Prospective risk of pancreatic cancer in familial pancreatic cancer kindreds. Cancer Res 2004;64:2634.

10. Klein AP, Beaty TH, Bailey-Wilson JE, et al. Evidence for a major gene influencing risk of pancreatic cancer. Genet Epidemiol 2002;23:133.

11. Hahn SA, Greenhalf B, Ellis I, et al. BRCA2 germline mutations in familial pancreatic carcinoma. J Natl Cancer Inst 2003;95:214.

12. Murphy KM, Brune KA, Griffin C, et al. Evaluation of candidate genes MAP2K4, MADH4, ACVR1B, and BRCA2 in familial pancreatic cancer: deleterious BRCA2 mutations in 17%. Cancer Res 2002;62:3789.

13. Roa BB, Boyd AA, Volcik K, et al. Ashkenazi Jewish population frequencies for common mutations in BRCA1 and BRCA2. Nat Genet 1996;14:185.

14. Couch FJ, Johnson MR, Rabe KG, et al. The prevalence of BRCA2 mutations in familial pancreatic cancer. Cancer Epidemiol Biomarkers Prev 2007;16:342.

15. Roberts NJ, Jiao Y, Yu J, et al. ATM mutations in patients with hereditary pancreatic cancer. Cancer Discov 2012;2:41.

16. Wang W, Chen S, Brune KA, et al. PancPRO: risk assessment for individuals with a family history of pancreatic cancer. J Clin Oncol 2007;25:1417.

17. van Lier MG, Wagner A, Mathus-Vliegen EM, et al. High cancer risk in Peutz-Jeghers syndrome: a systematic review and surveillance recommendations. Am J Gastroenterol 2010;105:1258.

18. Goldstein AM, Fraser MC, Struewing JP, et al. Increased risk of pancreatic cancer in melanoma-prone kindreds with p16INK4 mutations. N Engl J Med 1995; 333:970.

19. de Snoo FA, Bishop DT, Bergman W, et al. Increased risk of cancer other than melanoma in CDKN2A founder mutation (p16-Leiden)-positive melanoma families. Clin Cancer Res 2008;14:7151.

20. van Asperen CJ, Brohet RM, Meijers-Heijboer EJ, et al. Cancer risks in BRCA2 families: estimates for sites other than breast and ovary. J Med Genet 2005;42:711.

21. Mocci E, Milne RL, Méndez-Villamil EY, et al. Risk of pancreatic cancer in breast cancer families from the breast cancer family registry. Cancer Epidemiol Biomarkers Prev 2013;22:803.

22. Ferrone CR, Levine DA, Tang LH, et al. BRCA germline mutations in Jewish patients with pancreatic adenocarcinoma. J Clin Oncol 2009;27:433.

23. Lal G, Liu G, Schmocker B, et al. Inherited predisposition to pancreatic adenocarcinoma: role of family history and germ-line p16, BRCA1, and BRCA2 mutations. Cancer Res 2000;60:409.

24. Thompson D, Easton DF, Breast Cancer Linkage Consortium. Cancer incidence in BRCA1 mutation carriers. J Natl Cancer Inst 2002;94:1358.

25. Xia B, Sheng Q, Nakanishi K, et al. Control of BRCA2 cellular and clinical functions by a nuclear partner, PALB2. Mol Cell 2006;22:719.

26. Slater EP, Langer P, Niemczyk E, et al. PALB2 mutations in European familial pancreatic cancer families. Clin Genet 2010;78:490.

27. Jones S, Hruban RH, Kamiyama M, et al. Exomic sequencing identifies PALB2 as a pancreatic cancer susceptibility gene. Science 2009;324:217.

28. Canto MI, Harinck F, Hruban RH, et al. International Cancer of the Pancreas Screening (CAPS) Consortium summit on the management of patients with increased risk for familial pancreatic cancer. Gut 2013;62:339.

29. Kempers MJ, Kuiper RP, Ockeloen CW, et al. Risk of colorectal and endometrial cancers in EPCAM deletion-positive Lynch syndrome: a cohort study. Lancet Oncol 2011;12:49.
30. Vallee RB, Gee MA. Make room for dynein. Trends Cell Biol 1998;8:490.
31. Win AK, Lindor NM, Winship I, et al. Risks of colorectal and other cancers after endometrial cancer for women with Lynch syndrome. J Natl Cancer Inst 2013; 105:274.
32. Goggins M, Offerhaus GJ, Hilgers W, et al. Pancreatic adenocarcinomas with DNA replication errors (RER+) are associated with wild-type K-ras and characteristic histopathology. Poor differentiation, a syncytial growth pattern, and pushing borders suggest RER+. Am J Pathol 1998;152:1501.
33. Syngal S, Brand RE, Church JM, et al. ACG clinical guideline: genetic testing and management of hereditary gastrointestinal cancer syndromes. Am J Gastroenterol 2015;110:223.
34. Ruijs MW, Verhoef S, Rookus MA, et al. TP53 germline mutation testing in 180 families suspected of Li-Fraumeni syndrome: mutation detection rate and relative frequency of cancers in different familial phenotypes. J Med Genet 2010; 47:421.
35. Giardiello FM, Offerhaus GJ, Lee DH, et al. Increased risk of thyroid and pancreatic carcinoma in familial adenomatous polyposis. Gut 1993;34:1394.
36. Jasperson KW, Tuohy TM, Neklason DW, et al. Hereditary and familial colon cancer. Gastroenterology 2010;138:2044.
37. Geoffroy-Perez B, Janin N, Ossian K, et al. Cancer risk in heterozygotes for ataxia-telangiectasia. Int J Cancer 2001;93:288.
38. Teich N, Rosendahl J, Tóth M, et al. Mutations of human cationic trypsinogen (PRSS1) and chronic pancreatitis. Hum Mutat 2006;27:721.
39. Lowenfels AB, Maisonneuve P, DiMagno EP, et al. Hereditary pancreatitis and the risk of pancreatic cancer. International Hereditary Pancreatitis Study Group. J Natl Cancer Inst 1997;89:442.
40. Rulyak SJ, Lowenfels AB, Maisonneuve P, et al. Risk factors for the development of pancreatic cancer in familial pancreatic cancer kindreds. Gastroenterology 2003;124:1292.
41. Sibert JR. Hereditary pancreatitis in England and Wales. J Med Genet 1978; 15:189.
42. Hruban RH, Adsay NV, Albores-Saavedra J, et al. Pancreatic intraepithelial neoplasia: a new nomenclature and classification system for pancreatic duct lesions. Am J Surg Pathol 2001;25:579.
43. Shi C, Klein AP, Goggins M, et al. Increased prevalence of precursor lesions in familial pancreatic cancer patients. Clin Cancer Res 2009;15:7737.
44. Brune K, Abe T, Canto M, et al. Multifocal neoplastic precursor lesions associated with lobular atrophy of the pancreas in patients having a strong family history of pancreatic cancer. Am J Surg Pathol 2006;30:1067.
45. Canto MI, Hruban RH, Fishman EK, et al. Frequent detection of pancreatic lesions in asymptomatic high-risk individuals. Gastroenterology 2012;142:796.
46. Bartsch DK, Dietzel K, Bargello M, et al. Multiple small "imaging" branch-duct type intraductal papillary mucinous neoplasms (IPMNs) in familial pancreatic cancer: indicator for concomitant high grade pancreatic intraepithelial neoplasia? Fam Cancer 2013;12:89.
47. Fukukura Y, Fujiyoshi F, Sasaki M, et al. Pancreatic duct: morphologic evaluation with MR cholangiopancreatography after secretin stimulation. Radiology 2002; 222:674.

48. Aithal GP, Chen RY, Cunningham JT, et al. Accuracy of EUS for detection of intraductal papillary mucinous tumor of the pancreas. Gastrointest Endosc 2002; 56:701.
49. Brentnall TA, Bronner MP, Byrd DR, et al. Early diagnosis and treatment of pancreatic dysplasia in patients with a family history of pancreatic cancer. Ann Intern Med 1999;131:247.
50. Kelly KA, Bardeesy N, Anbazhagan R, et al. Targeted nanoparticles for imaging incipient pancreatic ductal adenocarcinoma. PLoS Med 2008;5:e85.
51. Topazian M, Enders F, Kimmey M, et al. Interobserver agreement for EUS findings in familial pancreatic-cancer kindreds. Gastrointest Endosc 2007;66:62.
52. Canto MI, Goggins M, Hruban RH, et al. Screening for early pancreatic neoplasia in high-risk individuals: a prospective controlled study. Clin Gastroenterol Hepatol 2006;4:766.
53. Wu J, Matthaei H, Maitra A, et al. Recurrent GNAS mutations define an unexpected pathway for pancreatic cyst development. Sci Transl Med 2011;3:92ra66.
54. Kanda M, Knight S, Topazian M, et al. Mutant GNAS detected in duodenal collections of secretin-stimulated pancreatic juice indicates the presence or emergence of pancreatic cysts. Gut 2013;62:1024.
55. Redston MS, Caldas C, Seymour AB, et al. p53 mutations in pancreatic carcinoma and evidence of common involvement of homocopolymer tracts in DNA microdeletions. Cancer Res 1994;54:3025.
56. Hruban RH, Goggins M, Parsons J, et al. Progression model for pancreatic cancer. Clin Cancer Res 2000;6:2969.
57. Kanda M, Sadakari Y, Borges M, et al. Mutant TP53 in duodenal samples of pancreatic juice from patients with pancreatic cancer or high-grade dysplasia. Clin Gastroenterol Hepatol 2013;11:719.

Advances in Surgical Management of Pancreatic Diseases

Jashodeep Datta, MD, Charles M. Vollmer Jr, MD*

KEYWORDS

- Surgery • Pancreas • Minimally invasive • Pancreatic cancer • Chronic pancreatitis
- Pancreatic fistula • Postoperative Morbidity Index • Pancreatic cystic neoplasm

KEY POINTS

- Preoperative risk stratification in pancreatic surgery allows rational selection of patients amenable for surgical therapy and prediction of postoperative morbidity.
- The Postoperative Morbidity Index is a novel tool that allows utility-based quantification of postoperative morbidity at the cohort level.
- Although minimally invasive pancreatectomy has been selectively applied at centers with expertise, there is insufficient evidence for its long-term equivalency or superiority compared with conventional open surgery.
- Borderline resectable pancreatic adenocarcinoma involves the regional mesenteric vasculature to a limited extent; resection for such tumors, although technically possible, is likely to result in positive surgical margins without preoperative therapy.
- The traditional paradigm of open pancreatic necrosectomy in infected pancreatic necrosis has been replaced by a surgical step-up approach, encompassing initial percutaneous drainage followed by minimally invasive approaches to necrosectomy.

INTRODUCTION

The surgical management of pancreatic diseases is rapidly evolving, encompassing advances in evidence-driven selection of patients amenable for surgical therapy, preoperative risk stratification, refinements in the technical conduct of pancreatic operations, and quantification of postoperative morbidity. These advances have resulted in dramatic reductions in mortality following pancreatic surgery over the last few

Disclosures: The authors have nothing to disclose.
Funding: None.
Division of Gastrointestinal Surgery, Department of Surgery, University of Pennsylvania Perelman School of Medicine, 3400 Spruce Street, Philadelphia, PA 19104, USA
* Corresponding author.
E-mail address: Charles.Vollmer@uphs.upenn.edu

decades, particularly at high-volume pancreatic centers.[1] Diagnosis, evaluation, and operative treatment of such patients are increasingly undertaken in a multidisciplinary format. Surgical decision making is complex and challenging, and requires an intimate understanding of disease pathobiology, host physiology, technical considerations, and evolving trends in the field. This article focuses on select key developments in the surgical management and perioperative principles associated with contemporary pancreatic surgery.

PREOPERATIVE RISK STRATIFICATION IN PANCREATIC SURGERY

Preoperative risk stratification has emerged as a critical decision-support tool in the pancreatic surgeon's skill set to estimate patients' risks of complications following pancreatectomy. This process is essential for patient-centered care, shared decision making with patients, and true informed consent. The ability to provide personalized risk estimates for patients undergoing pancreatectomy, or any other operation, has been revolutionized with the introduction of the American College of Surgeons (ACS) National Surgical Quality Improvement Project (NSQIP), which collects high-quality, standardized clinical data on preoperative risk factors and 22 rigorously defined postoperative complications from more than 500 hospitals in the United States.[2,3] Using this platform, a universal and procedure-specific risk calculator encompasses several preoperatively known variables (eg, age group, sex, steroid use, diabetes, smoking history, body mass index) to estimate a composite and complication-specific risk profile (http://www.riskcalculator.facs.org).[4]

This multi-institutional ACS-NSQIP data set has been used by several groups to develop risk prediction models capable of predicting postoperative morbidity and mortality following pancreaticoduodenectomy (PD)[5] and distal pancreatectomy (DP)[6]; the espoused benefits of these simple risk estimation systems include appropriate patient counseling and preoperative expectation management, allowing comparison of risk-adjusted outcomes between different institutions, and optimizing patient physiology before major pancreatectomy. However, these models are subject to limitations inherent in the ACS-NSQIP data set, including the inability to (1) determine pancreatectomy-specific complications (eg, delayed gastric emptying [DGE], postoperative pancreatic fistula [POPF], biliary leak/fistula), (2) ascertain complications beyond the 30-day accrual period, or (3) account for hospital-specific variations in pancreatic surgery volume and the corresponding impact on postoperative complications.[7]

Accordingly, a recently proposed preoperative risk prediction model for PD has drawn on multinational data from 4 high-volume European pancreatic centers. Aptly named the Preoperative Pancreatic Resection (PREPARE) score, this model effectively discriminated patients into low-risk, intermediate-risk, or high-risk for major complications (ie, Clavien-Dindo complication grades III and IV[8]) based on 5 physiologic variables (heart rate, systolic blood pressure, hemoglobin and albumin levels, American Society of Anesthesiologists [ASA] score) and 3 operative variables (whether surgery was elective or not, type of surgical procedure, and whether the origin of disease was pancreatic or not). Notably, this score accounted for clinically relevant POPF (CR-POPF), was not restricted to 30-day complication data, and prospectively validated the derived PREPARE score in 429 patients across the participating institutions.[9]

Recognizing the inability of the universal ACS-NSQIP registry to account for pancreatectomy-specific variables and effectively predict pancreatectomy-specific morbidity, the ACS has championed the initiation of a hepatopancreatobiliary (HPB)-centered module to better capture key outcomes in this population; the so-called Pancreatectomy Demonstration Project (PDP).[10] The ACS-NSQIP PDP encompasses intraoperative variables such as pancreatic duct size, gland texture, need for vascular resection, method of pancreatic (eg, pancreaticojejunostomy vs pancreaticogastrostomy) or intestinal (eg, gastrojejunostomy vs duodenojejunostomy) reconstruction, use of intraoperative drain placement (discussed later), and use of minimally invasive approaches, while also accruing pancreatectomy-specific complications such as DGE, POPF, and need for postoperative percutaneous drainage.[11–14] This initiative promises to improve large-scale prediction of pancreatectomy-specific complications, provide risk-adjusted registries with HPB-specific data, facilitate multi-institutional clinical trials, and augment the quality improvement initiatives already underway in pancreatic surgery. These and other currently used risk assessment and prognostic modeling systems in pancreatic surgery are comprehensively reviewed elsewhere.[15]

QUANTIFYING THE MORBIDITY OF POSTPANCREATECTOMY COMPLICATIONS

Beyond the preoperative prediction of postoperative morbidity, pancreatic surgeons can now provide a quantitative analysis of the impact of those complications on patients. Such a quantitative instrument could serve as a benchmark for surgical quality and standardize research analysis of pancreatic resections across institutions. The Postoperative Morbidity Index (PMI) is the first such effort in quantifying postoperative morbidity at the cohort level.[16] The PMI combines 2 highly validated, publicly available systems: (1) the Modified Accordion Classification System,[17] in which numerical severity weights were stringently established by expert opinion for each of 6 complication severity grades; and (2) the ACS-NSQIP, which provides a uniform method for skilled data experts to identify 22 rigorously defined perioperative complications. Each ACS-NSQIP complication is assigned a utility-based Accordion severity weight ranging from 0.110 (grade 1/mild) to 1.00 (grade 6/death). PMI equals the sum of complication severity weights (total burden) divided by total number of patients; it can range along the utility scale from 0 (ie, no complication in any patient) to 1.00 (ie, all patients died of complications). It provides a population-level measure of the morbidity of a procedure irrespective of whether a patient experienced a complication in the series. As such, higher PMIs denote populations with greater average morbidity.[18–20]

The utility of the PMI in the assessment of complications was first shown for 5 common abdominal operations performed at a single institution.[16] Subsequently, using a cohort derived from 9 high-volume pancreatic centers, the PMI of the 3 most common pancreatic resections (PD,[20] DP,[18] and total pancreatectomy [TP])[19] have been established. The PMI improves on the imprecision of nonspecific or qualitative complication grading (eg, Dindo-Clavien classification), and reflects not only the occurrence of complications but also their impact on patients.[19] Perhaps most importantly, the PMI establishes that complications of one type (eg, pulmonary embolism) may have varying impacts across the severity spectrum in different patients.

However, a notable limitation of these iterations of the PMI model is that it is not yet risk-adjusted; it is unable to account for changes in patients' physiologic makeup or processes of postpancreatectomy care over time.[19] Moreover, disparities in patient risk between surgeons and institutions reinforce the need for comprehensive risk-adjusted modeling when assessing the impact of procedure-specific complications. Accordingly, efforts are underway to refine the PMI metric in order to achieve such risk adjustment.

PANCREATIC FISTULA PREDICTION AND MITIGATION STRATEGIES

POPF, which results from pancreatointestinal anastomotic disruption/leakage following PD, is a dominant contributor to post-PD morbidity and is often lethal.[21]

Although overall outcomes following PD have improved dramatically over the years, POPF rates remain high (up to 33%).[22] Although several studies have identified risk factors that reproducibly predict POPF, comprehensive risk modeling has only recently been made possible with the advent of a universal classification scheme for POPF, proposed by the International Study Group of Pancreatic Fistula in 2005.[23] This classification establishes definitions that delineate between purely biochemical POPFs (grade A) and those deemed clinically relevant (grades B and C). This framework has allowed the identification of distinct risk factors (ie, gland texture, pathology, duct diameter, and intraoperative blood loss) that have been incorporated into a validated metric for the prediction of CR-POPF following PD, known as the Fistula Risk Score (FRS).[24–26] This novel decision-support tool offers a weighted approach that assigns quantitative values to the presence of the aforementioned risk factors (**Table 1**).

Beyond the prediction of CR-POPF per se, strategies to mitigate the incidence and impact of CR-POPF have been proposed, including anastomotic stents, prophylactic somatostatin analogue therapy, autologous tissue patches, and tissue sealants.[27] Intraoperative juxtapancreatic drain placement is another common management strategy. Despite claims that drains are unnecessary because of their association with higher rates of POPF,[28,29] a recent randomized, controlled trial indicated that routine elimination of drain use in PD increases the severity and frequency of overall complications, resulting in an unacceptably high mortality.[30] Drawing on this same randomized patient cohort, McMillan and colleagues[27] used the FRS as a risk assessment tool to determine the effect of intraoperative drain placement on the incidence of CR-POPF. Patients with negligible/low FRS risk had higher rates of CR-POPF when drains were used (14.8 vs 4.0%). In contrast, there were significantly fewer CR-POPFs (12.2 vs 29.5%) when drains were used with moderate/high FRS patients; these particular patients who had a CR-POPF also had reduced 90-day mortality when a drain was used. These data suggest that assessment of patient risk at the time of operative reconstruction may allow a more selective strategy of intraoperative

Table 1
FRS for the prediction of CR-POPF after pancreaticoduodenectomy

Risk Factor	Parameter	Points
Gland Texture	Firm	0
	Soft	2
Pathology	Pancreatic adenocarcinoma or pancreatitis	0
	Ampullary, duodenal, cystic, islet cell, and so forth	1
Pancreatic Duct Diameter (mm)	≥5	0
	4	1
	3	2
	2	3
	≤1	4
Intraoperative Blood Loss (mL)	≤400	0
	401–700	1
	701–1000	2
	>1000	3
		Total 0–10 points

From Callery MP, Pratt WB, Kent TS, et al. A prospectively validated clinical risk score accurately predicts pancreatic fistula after pancreatoduodenectomy. J Am Coll Surg 2013;216(1):6; with permission.

drain use, particularly in patients with negligible/low risk of CR-POPF development. Adoption of this strategy, along with targeted, early drain removal, has decreased the CR-POPF rate from 12% to 4% at our institution (101 patients over the last year, Vollmer et al, unpublished data, 2015). Moreover, beyond drain management, the FRS has been useful in understanding the impact of other operative and perioperative techniques used during pancreatectomy.[31,32]

EXPANDING INDICATIONS FOR RESECTION OF PANCREATIC CYSTIC NEOPLASMS

Pancreatic cystic neoplasms (PCN), including main-duct (MD) or branch-duct (BD) intraductal papillary mucinous neoplasms (IPMN) and mucinous cystic neoplasms (MCN), are increasingly detected, owing in part to liberal application of, and technological improvements in, cross-sectional imaging techniques. IPMNs and MCNs span a spectrum of neoplastic transformation, and recommendations for resection or surveillance of these lesions are typically based on the preoperative risk stratification proposed in consensus guidelines from the International Association of Pancreatology (IAP) in 2006 (Sendai criteria),[33] and updated in 2012 (Fukuoka criteria).[34] Per the Fukuoka guidelines, resection is recommended in all surgically fit patients with MD-IPMN and MCN. In MD-IPMN, if the resection margin is positive for high-grade dysplasia, additional resection should be attempted in order to obtain at least moderate-grade dysplasia. In MCN less than 4 cm without mural nodules, minimally invasive pancreatectomy (discussed later) or parenchyma-sparing resections and DP with splenic preservation could be considered.[34]

For management of BD-IPMN, the 2012 guidelines also outlined worrisome features and high-risk stigmata; clinicoradiographic characteristics that add nuance to surgical decision making beyond consideration of cyst size alone. For instance, a BD-IPMN greater than 3 cm without high-risk stigmata (ie, obstructive jaundice from a pancreatic head lesion, enhancing solid component within cyst, or main pancreatic duct >10 mm in size) can potentially be observed without immediate resection. If worrisome features (ie, pancreatitis, thickened/enhancing cyst walls, MD 5–9 mm, nonenhancing mural nodule, or abrupt change in pancreatic duct caliber with distal pancreatic atrophy) are present, BD-IPMNs should be evaluated with endoscopic ultrasonography (EUS). Findings of positive cytology, definite mural nodule, and/or suspected MD involvement on EUS should drive the decision to resect. Lack of these features on EUS instead warrants close surveillance with MRI and EUS every 3 to 6 months.[34]

It deserves mention that these criteria are not intended to supplant clinical judgment or patient preference. For instance, younger (<65 years) fit patients with cyst size greater than 2 cm and concerning imaging/pathologic features, who may not otherwise fit resection criteria, may be considered for surgery because of the cumulative risk of malignancy over their anticipated lifespan. In addition, recent evidence indicates that caution should be exercised when managing BD-IPMNs greater than 3 cm expectantly. In a single-institution retrospective review of 543 patients with BD-IPMN, Sahora and colleagues[35] showed that although the risk of high-grade dysplasia in nonworrisome lesions less than 3 cm was only 6.5%, the risk increased to nearly 10% when the size threshold was increased to greater than 3 cm, with 1 of those cases representing invasive carcinoma. The investigators concluded that although expectant management of BD-IPMN using the original Sendai criteria is likely safe, larger lesions may harbor incipient or frank malignancy, even in the absence of worrisome features. Another robust recent series from our institution confirms the 3-cm size cutoff as highly relevant.[36] Ultimately, a personalized approach to surgical resection of PCNs must entertain not only the risk of malignancy, presence of symptoms, and cyst size but also patient preferences; as such, balancing the risk of perioperative morbidity with the burden of prolonged surveillance is of utmost importance. Much remains to be achieved in establishing better, more precise prediction of the biological threat of these lesions. At select institutions, the management of PCNs occurs in a multidisciplinary group approach (so-called cyst clinic), similar to the manner in which pancreatic cancer is managed.

BORDERLINE RESECTABLE PANCREATIC DUCTAL ADENOCARCINOMA (PDAC)

There is growing recognition of borderline resectable PDAC as a distinct clinical entity, best conceptualized as tumors that involve the regional mesenteric vasculature (ie, superior mesenteric artery [SMA], common hepatic artery [CHA], superior mesenteric vein [SMV], and portal vein [PV]) to a limited extent; resection for such tumors, although technically possible, is likely to result in positive surgical margins (a highly negative prognosticator) without preoperative chemotherapy with or without radiotherapy (C ± RT).[37] Pioneering studies by the group from MD Anderson Cancer Center,[38] consensus guidelines from The Americas Hepatopancreatobiliary Association/Society for Surgery of the Alimentary Tract/Society of Surgical Oncology/National Comprehensive Care Network,[39,40] and more recently clinical trial protocols from the Alliance for Clinical Trials in Oncology Intergroup A021101 trial[37] have resulted in a contemporary definition for borderline resectable PDAC as localized tumors with 1 or more of the following: (1) interface between primary tumor and SMV-PV measuring greater than or equal to 180° of the circumference of the vein wall; (2) short-segment occlusion of the SMV-PV with normal vein above and below the level of obstruction that is amenable to resection and venous reconstruction; (3) short-segment interface (of any degree) between tumor and CHA with normal artery proximal and distal to the interface that is amenable to resection and arterial reconstruction; (4) an interface between the tumor and SMA/celiac trunk measuring less than 180° of the circumference of the artery wall.[37] Recently, an international consensus statement on this entity has also been derived.[41]

Surgical considerations for this disease entity have also evolved with growing understanding of its natural history; key elements of surgical decision making in this regard deserve mention. First, although margin-negative resection of the primary tumor (and its draining nodal basin) is critical, it is increasingly difficult to achieve de novo with increasing involvement of the major vascular structures. In this regard, rational application of preoperative C ± RT may select for patients with favorable tumor biology, and host physiology, who are most likely to benefit from aggressive local resection; by the same token, patients with rapid progression are spared the morbidity of major pancreatectomy. Second, in the cohort of carefully selected patients who complete preoperative therapy without progression (or perhaps tumor regression; so-called downstaging), aggressive surgical extirpation, with or without vascular resection, seems to be of benefit. Emerging data indicate that resection of the SMV-PV and CHA at the time of pancreatectomy is associated with acceptable perioperative morbidity and mortality[42]; however, SMA resection and/or reconstruction seems futile.[43,44] In addition, lack of sensitivity of radiographic staging (ie, Response Evaluation Criteria in Solid Tumors [RECIST]) seems to undercut the true efficacy of neoadjuvant C ± RT.[45] A recent single-institution study revealed that only 12% of 129 patients with borderline resectable PDAC had RECIST partial response, whereas only 1 patient (0.8%) was downstaged to resectable status, following neoadjuvant chemoradiotherapy. Despite these unfavorable radiographic indicators, R0 resection was possible in 66% of patients.[46]

In addition to standardization of radiographic and surgical criteria for resection, a multidisciplinary approach is critical to accurately determine the impact of preoperative therapy on borderline resectable PDAC and outcomes thereof; mechanisms to standardize these components (eg, surgical technique, chemotherapy regimens, radiotherapy field design) have been incorporated into the Intergroup A021101 trial, results from which are eagerly awaited. Notwithstanding, at this time there is no high-level evidence to support that neoadjuvant therapy for pancreatic cancer offers a survival benefit for either resectable or borderline resectable disease. This topic will continue to be a fertile, and necessary, area for future investigation and will mandate scrupulous study designs.

MINIMALLY INVASIVE PANCREATIC RESECTION

The advent of minimally invasive approaches (ie, laparoscopic or robotic-assisted laparoscopic) has revolutionized the surgical treatment of many benign and malignant conditions. Although initially sluggish, minimally invasive pancreatectomy (MIP) is increasingly gaining acceptance, particularly at specialized high-volume pancreatic centers. Although skeptics of MIP question the ability of these approaches to maintain oncologic integrity, proponents cite potential advantages associated with laparoscopy: (1) decreased inflammatory responses with less perioperative immunosuppression, which may translate into potential oncologic benefit[47]; (2) improved visualization (particularly with a robotic-assisted approach) and magnified view allowing more precise dissection; and (3) advanced degrees of freedom of technical maneuvers.[48] Controversy persists regarding efficacy of MIP versus open pancreatectomy, as well as which MIP platform is optimal.

The use of minimally invasive DP is increasing in surgical practice, with recent literature showing several benefits compared with its open counterpart.[48] Although adequately powered randomized trials comparing minimally invasive versus open DP are not currently available, several large retrospective comparative series have shown the feasibility, safety, and favorable outcomes associated with this approach.[49–51] Venkat and colleagues[49] performed a systematic review of 18 such studies, including 1814 patients (43% laparoscopic, 57% open). Although long-term oncologic outcomes could not be assessed, the laparoscopic approach was associated with equivalent rates of margin positivity, as well as decreased intraoperative blood loss, overall complications, surgical site infections, and duration of postoperative stay compared with an open approach. In a population-based cohort of 8957 patients from the National Inpatient Sample undergoing DP, just 382 (4.3%) underwent minimally invasive DP, indicating its relative lack of use thus far. On multivariable analysis, minimally invasive DP was associated with fewer overall complications and postoperative infections, as well as shorter duration of stay; no differences in rates of in-hospital mortality, concomitant splenectomy, or total costs were observed.[51] A recent single-institution experience suggested that robotic assistance for laparoscopic DP decreases the risk of conversion to an open resection, while maintaining equivalent outcomes compared with a purely laparoscopic approach; the investigators concluded that robotic assistance may broaden indications for minimally invasive DP, particularly for cancer.[50]

In contrast with minimally invasive DP, minimally invasive PD (MIPD) continues to lack widespread acceptance because long-term oncologic outcomes comparing MIPD with the open approach are lacking.[48] Although short-term outcomes (ie, duration of stay, blood loss, overall and pancreas-specific complications) seemed comparable with those achieved with the open approach when highly skilled specialists applied MIPD techniques (**Table 2**),[52,53,56] the intentional patient selection bias

Table 2
Selected series of minimally invasive PD reporting outcomes for at least 50 patients

Publication, Year	Patients (n)	Approach	Operative Time (min)	EBL (mL)	CR-POPF	DGE	LOS (d)	Mortality (%)
Palanivelu et al,[52] 2009	75	Lap	357	74	7	NR	8	1.3
Kendrick et al,[53] 2010	62	Lap	368	240	18	15	7	1.6
Giulianotti et al,[54] 2010	60	Robotic	421	394	21	5	22	3
Kim et al,[55] 2012	100	Lap	487	NR	6	2	20	1
Asbun et al,[56] 2012	53	Lap	541	195	10	11	8	6
Zeh et al,[57] 2012	50	Robotic	568	350	20	20	10	2
Zureikat et al,[58] 2013	132	Robotic	527	300	7	NR	10	1.5

Abbreviations: EBL, median estimated blood loss; Lap, laparoscopic; LOS, length of stay.

inherent in these early experiences limit assessment of equivalency or superiority of MIPD. Moreover, in addition to the technical complexity associated with MIPD,[48] there is no definitive evidence indicating that earlier postoperative recovery following MIPD mitigates the major morbidity of the operation or allows more timely initiation of adjuvant therapy. Based on existing data, it is therefore uncertain whether MIPD offers a substantial advantage compared with open PD beyond possibly restoring the functional capacity of patients to their premorbid states more rapidly. Moreover, significant concerns remain about the ability to generalize from these minimally invasive approaches given the lengthy learning curves necessary for proficiency (ie, as many as 250 cases).[58] Longitudinal follow-up and carefully controlled studies are needed to ascertain whether MIPD will remain a niche practice or garner broader adoption.

MINIMALLY INVASIVE PARADIGM FOR SURGICAL MANAGEMENT OF INFECTED PANCREATIC NECROSIS

Although most (~80%) patients with acute pancreatitis experience resolution of symptoms, the remainder progress to a more complicated course characterized by necrotizing pancreatitis with or without associated organ failure.[59] Approximately 30% of patients with necrotizing pancreatitis develop infected necrosis,[60] with in-hospital mortalities approaching 40% if organ failure ensues.[61] In general, although sterile asymptomatic pancreatic necrosis can be treated with supportive management, infected pancreatic necrosis remains a near-absolute indication for invasive intervention. Barring impending intra-abdominal sepsis and hemodynamic collapse, pancreatic necrosectomy in clinically stable patients, performed via open or minimally invasive approaches, should be postponed until the necrosis appears radiographically walled off; this typically correlates with an observation period of 4 to 6 weeks.[62]

The traditional paradigm of mandatory open pancreatic necrosectomy in infected necrosis has been replaced by a surgical step-up approach, championed in the randomized PANTER (PAncreatitis, Necrosectomy versus sTEp up appRoach) trial conducted by the Dutch Pancreatitis Study Group.[63] In this study, 88 patients were randomly allocated to either maximal necrosectomy via laparotomy (n = 45) or percutaneous catheter drainage (PCD) followed, if necessary, by video-assisted retroperitoneal debridement (VARD; n = 43). Both procedures were followed by continuous peritoneal lavage. The composite end point of major complications and/or death was observed less frequently in the step-up compared with the open necrosectomy cohort (40% vs 69%; $P = .006$).[63] In light of this groundbreaking study, PCD via a retroperitoneal and transperitoneal route is now considered the initial step in the contemporary treatment of infected necrosis per IAP/American Pancreatic Association consensus guidelines; drainage of purulent material under pressure mitigates ongoing sepsis and may postpone or even obviate necrosectomy (in up to 50% of patients). In some cases, drainage alone (without additive interventions) may suffice.[64]

If PCD fails, an array of minimally invasive options for necrosectomy has emerged, with growing evidence supporting their superiority to open necrosectomy with respect to procedural complications and resource use. These options include sinus tract necrosectomy, VARD, retroperitoneoscopic necrosectomy, endoscopic transluminal drainage and necrosectomy, and laparoscopic transgastric necrosectomy.[65] VARD, the best studied of these options, involves removal of loosely adherent and visible necrosis under videoscopic guidance from a left-sided retroperitoneal approach, wide catheter drainage, and postoperative lavage until the effluent is clear.[66] In a multicenter prospective cohort study by Horvath and colleagues,[67] VARD was technically feasible in 60% of patients requiring necrosectomy (ie, failing PCD alone), was associated with a favorable complication profile compared historically with open necrosectomy (6% hemorrhage, 10% enteric fistulas), and did not result in any mortalities. However, 16 of 31 patients (52%) requiring necrosectomy ultimately underwent open necrosectomy because of the presence of a centromedial peripancreatic collection with inferior extension into the mesenteric root; a significant negative predictor for successful VARD.

A minimally invasive alternative to VARD is endoscopic transluminal drainage/ necrosectomy, particularly if the infectious nidus lies in close proximity to the gastric or duodenal lumen. The peripancreatic collection is accessed via EUS guidance, and serially dilated with balloon dilators; fully covered self-expandable metallic stents may be used to reinforce the fistula tract. Once access is gained, necrosectomy may be performed with various instruments (eg, snares, nets, baskets).[65] Typically, multiple attempts are required for complete debridement. A pilot randomized trial (PENGUIN [Pancreatitis Endoscopic Transgastric vs Primary Necrosectomy in Patients with Infected Pancreatic Necrosis]) in 22 patients comparing endoscopic necrosectomy with VARD suggested an attenuated proinflammatory postprocedure response (measure by systemic interleukin-6 levels) and lower rates of complications/death in the endoscopic cohort.[68] To validate this question on a larger scale, the Dutch multicenter TENSION (Transluminal endoscopic step-up approach versus minimally invasive surgical step-up approach in patients with infected necrotising pancreatitis) trial (SRCTN09186711) is randomizing patients to either endoscopic transluminal drainage (if necessary) followed by (if necessary) endoscopic necrosectomy versus PCD followed by (if necessary) VARD. The primary end point is a composite of major complications and death.[69]

A recently proposed novel surgical option is laparoscopic transgastric necrosectomy, which uses 2 to 3 laparoscopic ports to achieve necrosectomy via a wide cyst-gastrostomy cavity. A retrospective report of 21 patients from Worhunsky and colleagues[70] revealed that complete debridement in a single operation was possible in almost all cases; more importantly, none of the patients required additional surgery, developed pancreatic/enteric fistulae, or experienced wound complications. Larger-scale studies comparing this and other minimally invasive techniques are planned, and will inform best practices in this rapidly evolving arena of pancreatic surgery.

EMERGING SURGICAL OPTIONS FOR THE MANAGEMENT OF CHRONIC PANCREATITIS

The irreversible process of chronic pancreatitis (CP) results in intractable pain, progressive endocrine and exocrine insufficiency, and (in a minority of patients) PDAC. Surgical management of CP must be tailored to the unique anatomic determinants of disease, encompassing (1) drainage procedures (ie, longitudinal pancreatojejunostomy) in patients with pancreatic ductal dilatation with (Frey procedure) or without (Puestow procedure) pancreatic head involvement; (2) formal resections in localized disease with small duct pancreatitis (eg, Whipple PD, Beger duodenum-sparing pancreatic head resection, or DP); and (3) total pancreatectomy with or without autoislet transplantation (TP-AIT).[71] Consensus guidelines indicate that TP-AIT is indicated for the treatment of intractable pain in patients with impaired quality of life (QOL) caused by CP (or recurrent acute pancreatitis) in whom medical, endoscopic, or prior surgical therapy have failed.[72] Patients with known genetic predisposition to CP (eg, hereditary pancreatitis caused by mutations in *PRSS1*, *SPINK1*, or *CFTR* genes) are given particular consideration for TP-AIT because of the low likelihood of disease remission.[72] Although TP removes the pancreatic parenchyma responsible for the pain, inflammation, and eventual cancer risk associated with CP, AIT prevents the brittle pancreatogenic diabetes associated with loss of both insulin and counter-regulatory glucagon. However, the primary objective of TP-AIT is mitigation of pain; diabetes control is a secondary goal.[72]

The operation involves resection of the entire pancreas, duodenum, distal common bile duct, and spleen (typically). Complete pancreatic mobilization is undertaken before ligation of the major blood supply (ie, gastroduodenal artery, splenic artery) in order to minimize warm ischemia time to the pancreatic islet cells. Following resection, the specimen is placed in cold preservation solution before transportation to a Good Medical Practice facility for islet processing; biliary and enteric reconstruction is performed during islet processing. Islet isolates are typically infused through the portal vein with engraftment in the liver. If high portal pressures (>25 cm H_2O) are detected, alternative sites of islet autotransplantation are sought (eg, intraperitoneal, gastric submucosa, beneath the renal capsule).[73,74]

The University of Minnesota experience of 409 consecutive patients with CP largely informs the growing understanding of the ramifications following TP-AIT. A majority (74%) of patients was female, almost all had narcotic-dependent pain before surgery, and 21% had undergone previous pancreatic resections. Following TP-AIT, actuarial survival was greater than 95% at 1 year and greater than 90% at 5 years. AIT function was achieved in 90% of patients, and 63% were independent of, or partially dependent on, exogenous insulin. Most importantly, 85% of patients experienced improvements in pain control postoperatively, with 59% ceasing narcotic use at 2 years. In Short Form 36 QOL surveys, significant improvements in all dimensions of physical and mental functioning were observed, whether patients were on narcotics or not.[74] Accumulating experience with TP-AIT is allowing optimization of patient selection and evidence-driven expansion of eligibility criteria for TP-IAT, which may improve recipients' endocrine function, pain relief, and QOL. Ongoing efforts to improve islet processing and engraftment, better understand the immunobiology of IAT, and optimize perioperative management will further contribute to enhanced postoperative outcomes for patients with CP in the future. Notwithstanding, it should be emphasized that this operation remains infrequently indicated and performed, with just a few centers in the United States performing more than 10 procedures a year. Its efficacy remains highly controversial.

SUMMARY

The ability to predict and prevent perioperative morbidity, gain access to the abdominal cavity and perform complex gastrointestinal reconstruction using endoscopic/laparoscopic techniques, and judiciously select patients with malignant and premalignant diseases who might benefit most from aggressive surgical resection are just a few of the major advances in pancreatic surgery that have taken the field to new levels. Technical advancements, as well as increasingly specialized training, have made pancreatic surgery safer, quicker, and more effective. Other technological advances being investigated are irreversible electroporation for pancreatic resection margin accentuation[75] and fluorescence-guided surgery to enhance intraoperative margin detection.[76,77] Centralization of multimodality pancreatic care to specialized centers of excellence allows a multidisciplinary approach to pancreatic diseases, resulting in improved outcomes with an emphasis on quality of delivered care. However, despite the aforementioned progress, there remains considerable room for improvement; for instance, 5-year survival for resectable PDAC remains approximately 20%. The growing understanding of the molecular and immunologic underpinnings of pancreatic disease, specifically cancer, will enable a more sophisticated approach to patient selection, disease detection, and surgical decision making in the near future.

REFERENCES

1. Lewis R, Drebin JA, Callery MP, et al. A contemporary analysis of survival for resected pancreatic ductal adenocarcinoma. HPB (Oxford) 2013;15(1):49–60.
2. Hall BL, Hamilton BH, Richards K, et al. Does surgical quality improve in the American College of Surgeons National Surgical Quality Improvement Program: an evaluation of all participating hospitals. Ann Surg 2009;250(3):363–76.
3. Ingraham AM, Richards KE, Hall BL, et al. Quality improvement in surgery: the American College of Surgeons National Surgical Quality Improvement Program approach. Adv Surg 2010;44:251–67.
4. Bilimoria KY, Liu Y, Paruch JL, et al. Development and evaluation of the universal ACS NSQIP surgical risk calculator: a decision aid and informed consent tool for patients and surgeons. J Am Coll Surg 2013;217(5):833–42.e1-3.
5. Greenblatt DY, Kelly KJ, Rajamanickam V, et al. Preoperative factors predict perioperative morbidity and mortality after pancreaticoduodenectomy. Ann Surg Oncol 2011;18(8):2126–35.
6. Kelly KJ, Greenblatt DY, Wan Y, et al. Risk stratification for distal pancreatectomy utilizing ACS-NSQIP: preoperative factors predict morbidity and mortality. J Gastrointest Surg 2011;15(2):250–9.
7. Epelboym I, Gawlas I, Lee JA, et al. Limitations of ACS-NSQIP in reporting complications for patients undergoing pancreatectomy: underscoring the need for a pancreas-specific module. World J Surg 2014;38(6):1461–7.
8. Dindo D, Demartines N, Clavien PA. Classification of surgical complications: a new proposal with evaluation in a cohort of 6336 patients and results of a survey. Ann Surg 2004;240(2):205–13.
9. Uzunoglu FG, Reeh M, Vettorazzi E, et al. Preoperative Pancreatic Resection (PREPARE) score: a prospective multicenter-based morbidity risk score. Ann Surg 2014;260(5):857–63.
10. Pitt HA, Kilbane M, Strasberg SM, et al. ACS-NSQIP has the potential to create an HPB-NSQIP option. HPB (Oxford) 2009;11(5):405–13.
11. Parmar AD, Sheffield KM, Vargas GM, et al. Factors associated with delayed gastric emptying after pancreaticoduodenectomy. HPB (Oxford) 2013;15(10):763–72.
12. Lee CW, Pitt HA, Riall TS, et al. Low drain fluid amylase predicts absence of pancreatic fistula following pancreatectomy. J Gastrointest Surg 2014;18(11): 1902–10.
13. Behrman SW, Zarzaur BL, Parmar A, et al. Routine drainage of the operative bed following elective distal pancreatectomy does not reduce the occurrence of complications. J Gastrointest Surg 2015;19(1):72–9 [discussion: 79].
14. Cooper AB, Parmar AD, Riall TS, et al. Does the use of neoadjuvant therapy for pancreatic adenocarcinoma increase postoperative morbidity and mortality rates? J Gastrointest Surg 2015;19(1):80–6 [discussion: 86–7].
15. Lewis RS Jr, Vollmer CM Jr. Risk scores and prognostic models in surgery: pancreas resection as a paradigm. Curr Probl Surg 2012;49(12):731–95.
16. Strasberg SM, Hall BL. Postoperative morbidity index: a quantitative measure of severity of postoperative complications. J Am Coll Surg 2011;213(5):616–26.
17. Porembka MR, Hall BL, Hirbe M, et al. Quantitative weighting of postoperative complications based on the Accordion Severity Grading System: demonstration of potential impact using the American College of Surgeons National Surgical Quality Improvement Program. J Am Coll Surg 2010;210(3):286–98.
18. Lee MK 4th, Lewis RS, Strasberg SM, et al. Defining the post-operative morbidity index for distal pancreatectomy. HPB (Oxford) 2014;16(10):915–23.

19. Datta J, Lewis RS Jr, Strasberg SM, et al. Quantifying the burden of complications following total pancreatectomy using the postoperative morbidity index: a multi-institutional perspective. J Gastrointest Surg 2015;19(3):506–15.
20. Vollmer CM Jr, Lewis RS, Hall BL, et al. Establishing a quantitative benchmark for morbidity in pancreatoduodenectomy using ACS-NSQIP, the Accordion Severity Grading System, and the Postoperative Morbidity Index. Ann Surg 2015;261(3):527–36.
21. McMillan MT, Vollmer CM Jr. Predictive factors for pancreatic fistula following pancreatectomy. Langenbecks Arch Surg 2014;399(7):811–24.
22. Pratt WB, Callery MP, Vollmer CM Jr. Risk prediction for development of pancreatic fistula using the ISGPF classification scheme. World J Surg 2008;32(3):419–28.
23. Bassi C, Dervenis C, Butturini G, et al. Postoperative pancreatic fistula: an international study group (ISGPF) definition. Surgery 2005;138(1):8–13.
24. Callery MP, Pratt WB, Kent TS, et al. A prospectively validated clinical risk score accurately predicts pancreatic fistula after pancreatoduodenectomy. J Am Coll Surg 2013;216(1):1–14.
25. Miller BC, Christein JD, Behrman SW, et al. A multi-institutional external validation of the fistula risk score for pancreatoduodenectomy. J Gastrointest Surg 2014;18(1):172–9.
26. McMillan MT, Vollmer CM Jr, Asbun HJ, et al. The characterization and prediction of ISGPF grade C fistulas following pancreatoduodenectomy. J Gastrointest Surg 2015. [Epub ahead of print].
27. McMillan MT, Fisher WE, Van Buren G 2nd, et al. The value of drains as a fistula mitigation strategy for pancreatoduodenectomy: something for everyone? Results of a randomized prospective multi-institutional study. J Gastrointest Surg 2015;19(1):21–30.
28. Conlon KC, Labow D, Leung D, et al. Prospective randomized clinical trial of the value of intraperitoneal drainage after pancreatic resection. Ann Surg 2001;234(4):487–93.
29. Correa-Gallego C, Brennan MF, D'Angelica M, et al. Operative drainage following pancreatic resection: analysis of 1122 patients resected over 5 years at a single institution. Ann Surg 2013;258(6):1051–8.
30. Van Buren G 2nd, Bloomston M, Hughes SJ, et al. A randomized prospective multicenter trial of pancreaticoduodenectomy with and without routine intraperitoneal drainage. Ann Surg 2014;259(4):605–12.
31. Sachs TE, Pratt WB, Kent TS, et al. The pancreaticojejunal anastomotic stent: friend or foe? Surgery 2013;153(5):651–62.
32. McMillan MT, Christein JD, Callery MP, et al. Prophylactic octreotide for pancreatoduodenectomy: more harm than good? HPB (Oxford) 2014;16(10):954–62.
33. Tanaka M, Chari S, Adsay V, et al. International consensus guidelines for management of intraductal papillary mucinous neoplasms and mucinous cystic neoplasms of the pancreas. Pancreatology 2006;6(1–2):17–32.
34. Tanaka M, Fernandez-del Castillo C, Adsay V, et al. International consensus guidelines 2012 for the management of IPMN and MCN of the pancreas. Pancreatology 2012;12(3):183–97.
35. Sahora K, Mino-Kenudson M, Brugge W, et al. Branch duct intraductal papillary mucinous neoplasms: does cyst size change the tip of the scale? A critical analysis of the revised international consensus guidelines in a large single-institutional series. Ann Surg 2013;258(3):466–75.

36. Hoffman RL, Gates JL, Kochman ML, et al. Analysis of cyst size and tumor markers in the management of pancreatic cysts: support for the original Sendai criteria. J Am Coll Surg 2015;220(6):1087–95.
37. Katz MH, Marsh R, Herman JM, et al. Borderline resectable pancreatic cancer: need for standardization and methods for optimal clinical trial design. Ann Surg Oncol 2013;20(8):2787–95.
38. Varadhachary GR, Tamm EP, Abbruzzese JL, et al. Borderline resectable pancreatic cancer: definitions, management, and role of preoperative therapy. Ann Surg Oncol 2006;13(8):1035–46.
39. Callery MP, Chang KJ, Fishman EK, et al. Pretreatment assessment of resectable and borderline resectable pancreatic cancer: expert consensus statement. Ann Surg Oncol 2009;16(7):1727–33.
40. Tempero MA, Malafa MP, Behrman SW, et al. Pancreatic adenocarcinoma, version 2.2014: featured updates to the NCCN guidelines. J Natl Compr Canc Netw 2014;12(8):1083–93.
41. Bockhorn M, Uzunoglu FG, Adham M, et al. Borderline resectable pancreatic cancer: a consensus statement by the International Study Group of Pancreatic Surgery (ISGPS). Surgery 2014;155(6):977–88.
42. Tseng JF, Raut CP, Lee JE, et al. Pancreaticoduodenectomy with vascular resection: margin status and survival duration. J Gastrointest Surg 2004;8(8):935–49.
43. Stitzenberg KB, Watson JC, Roberts A, et al. Survival after pancreatectomy with major arterial resection and reconstruction. Ann Surg Oncol 2008;15(5):1399–406.
44. Mollberg N, Rahbari NN, Koch M, et al. Arterial resection during pancreatectomy for pancreatic cancer: a systematic review and meta-analysis. Ann Surg 2011;254(6):882–93.
45. Lopez NE, Prendergast C, Lowy AM. Borderline resectable pancreatic cancer: definitions and management. World J Gastroenterol 2014;20(31):10740–51.
46. Katz MH, Fleming JB, Bhosale P, et al. Response of borderline resectable pancreatic cancer to neoadjuvant therapy is not reflected by radiographic indicators. Cancer 2012;118(23):5749–56.
47. Carter JJ, Whelan RL. The immunologic consequences of laparoscopy in oncology. Surg Oncol Clin N Am 2001;10(3):655–77.
48. Stauffer JA, Asbun HJ. Minimally invasive pancreatic surgery. Semin Oncol 2015;42(1):123–33.
49. Venkat R, Edil BH, Schulick RD, et al. Laparoscopic distal pancreatectomy is associated with significantly less overall morbidity compared to the open technique: a systematic review and meta-analysis. Ann Surg 2012;255(6):1048–59.
50. Daouadi M, Zureikat AH, Zenati MS, et al. Robot-assisted minimally invasive distal pancreatectomy is superior to the laparoscopic technique. Ann Surg 2013;257(1):128–32.
51. Tran Cao HS, Lopez N, Chang DC, et al. Improved perioperative outcomes with minimally invasive distal pancreatectomy: results from a population-based analysis. JAMA Surg 2014;149(3):237–43.
52. Palanivelu C, Rajan PS, Rangarajan M, et al. Evolution in techniques of laparoscopic pancreaticoduodenectomy: a decade long experience from a tertiary center. J Hepatobiliary Pancreat Surg 2009;16(6):731–40.
53. Kendrick ML, Cusati D. Total laparoscopic pancreaticoduodenectomy: feasibility and outcome in an early experience. Arch Surg 2010;145(1):19–23.
54. Giulianotti PC, Sbrana F, Bianco FM, et al. Robot-assisted laparoscopic pancreatic surgery: single-surgeon experience. Surg Endosc 2010;24:1646–57.

55. Kim SC, Song KB, Jung YS, et al. Short-term clinical outcomes for 100 consecutive cases of laparoscopic pylorus-preserving pancreatoduodenectomy: improvement with surgical experience. Surg Endosc 2013;27:95–103.

56. Asbun HJ, Stauffer JA. Laparoscopic vs open pancreaticoduodenectomy: overall outcomes and severity of complications using the Accordion Severity Grading System. J Am Coll Surg 2012;215(6):810–9.

57. Zeh HJ, Zureikat AH, Secrest A, et al. Outcomes after robot-assisted pancreaticoduodenectomy for periampullary lesions. Ann Surg Oncol 2012;19:864–70.

58. Zureikat AH, Moser AJ, Boone BA, et al. 250 robotic pancreatic resections: safety and feasibility. Ann Surg 2013;258(4):554–9 [discussion: 559–62].

59. Banks PA, Bollen TL, Dervenis C, et al. Classification of acute pancreatitis–2012: revision of the Atlanta classification and definitions by international consensus. Gut 2013;62(1):102–11.

60. van Santvoort HC, Bakker OJ, Bollen TL, et al. A conservative and minimally invasive approach to necrotizing pancreatitis improves outcome. Gastroenterology 2011;141(4):1254–63.

61. Petrov MS, Shanbhag S, Chakraborty M, et al. Organ failure and infection of pancreatic necrosis as determinants of mortality in patients with acute pancreatitis. Gastroenterology 2010;139(3):813–20.

62. Besselink MG, Verwer TJ, Schoenmaeckers EJ, et al. Timing of surgical intervention in necrotizing pancreatitis. Arch Surg 2007;142(12):1194–201.

63. van Santvoort HC, Besselink MG, Bakker OJ, et al. A step-up approach or open necrosectomy for necrotizing pancreatitis. N Engl J Med 2010;362(16):1491–502.

64. Working Group IAP/APA Acute Pancreatitis Guidelines. IAP/APA evidence-based guidelines for the management of acute pancreatitis. Pancreatology 2013;13(4 Suppl 2):e1–15.

65. Hollemans RA, van Brunschot S, Bakker OJ, et al. Minimally invasive intervention for infected necrosis in acute pancreatitis. Expert Rev Med Devices 2014;11(6): 637–48.

66. van Santvoort HC, Besselink MG, Horvath KD, et al. Videoscopic assisted retroperitoneal debridement in infected necrotizing pancreatitis. HPB (Oxford) 2007; 9(2):156–9.

67. Horvath K, Freeny P, Escallon J, et al. Safety and efficacy of video-assisted retroperitoneal debridement for infected pancreatic collections: a multicenter, prospective, single-arm phase 2 study. Arch Surg 2010;145(9):817–25.

68. Bakker OJ, van Santvoort HC, van Brunschot S, et al. Endoscopic transgastric vs surgical necrosectomy for infected necrotizing pancreatitis: a randomized trial. JAMA 2012;307(10):1053–61.

69. van Brunschot S, van Grinsven J, Voermans RP, et al. Transluminal endoscopic step-up approach versus minimally invasive surgical step-up approach in patients with infected necrotising pancreatitis (TENSION trial): design and rationale of a randomised controlled multicenter trial [ISRCTN09186711]. BMC Gastroenterol 2013;13:161.

70. Worhunsky DJ, Qadan M, Dua MM, et al. Laparoscopic transgastric necrosectomy for the management of pancreatic necrosis. J Am Coll Surg 2014;219(4): 735–43.

71. Ni Q, Yun L, Roy M, et al. Advances in surgical treatment of chronic pancreatitis. World J Surg Oncol 2015;13:34.

72. Bellin MD, Freeman ML, Gelrud A, et al. Total pancreatectomy and islet autotransplantation in chronic pancreatitis: recommendations from PancreasFest. Pancreatology 2014;14(1):27–35.

73. Blondet JJ, Carlson AM, Kobayashi T, et al. The role of total pancreatectomy and islet autotransplantation for chronic pancreatitis. Surg Clin North Am 2007;87(6): 1477–501, x.

74. Sutherland DE, Radosevich DM, Bellin MD, et al. Total pancreatectomy and islet autotransplantation for chronic pancreatitis. J Am Coll Surg 2012;214(4): 409–24.

75. Martin RC 2nd, Kwon D, Chalikonda S, et al. Treatment of 200 locally advanced (stage III) pancreatic adenocarcinoma patients with irreversible electroporation: safety and efficacy. Ann Surg 2015;262(3):486–94.

76. Hiroshima Y, Maawy A, Zhang Y, et al. Fluorescence-guided surgery in combination with UVC irradiation cures metastatic human pancreatic cancer in orthotopic mouse models. PLoS One 2014;9(6):e99977.

77. Metildi CA, Kaushal S, Pu M, et al. Fluorescence-guided surgery with a fluorophore-conjugated antibody to carcinoembryonic antigen (CEA), that highlights the tumor, improves surgical resection and increases survival in orthotopic mouse models of human pancreatic cancer. Ann Surg Oncol 2014;21(4): 1405–11.

Pancreas Transplantation in the Modern Era

Robert R. Redfield, MD[a],*, Michael R. Rickels, MD, MS[b], Ali Naji, MD, PhD[c], Jon S. Odorico, MD[a]

KEYWORDS

- Pancreas transplantation • Islet transplantation • Diabetes • Pancreas diseases
- Outcomes

KEY POINTS

- The field of pancreas transplantation has evolved from an experimental procedure in the 1980s to become a routine transplant in the modern era.
- With outcomes continuing to improve and the significant mortality, quality-of-life and end-organ disease benefits, pancreas transplantation should be offered to more patients.
- In this paper, we review current indications, patient selection, surgical considerations, complications, and outcomes in the modern era of pancreas transplantation.

TRADITIONAL INDICATIONS FOR PANCREAS TRANSPLANTATION

Type 1 diabetes mellitus (T1DM) is the traditional indication for pancreas transplantation. Caused by autoimmune destruction of the insulin-producing β-cells contained in the endocrine islets of the pancreas, T1DM is a disease of insulin deficiency that ultimately progresses to loss of all physiologic insulin secretion. The prevalence of T1DM in the United States is estimated to be 1,250,000 individuals, and the annual incidence of 35,000 new cases diagnosed is increasing each year. Patients are dependent on intensive insulin therapy delivered by multiple daily injections

[a] Division of Transplantation, Department of Surgery, University of Wisconsin School of Medicine and Public Health, 600 Highland Avenue, Clinical Science Cntr-H4/772, Madison, WI 53792, USA; [b] Division of Endocrinology, Diabetes & Metabolism, Department of Medicine, University of Pennsylvania Perelman School of Medicine, 2-134 Smilow Center for Translational Research, 3400 Civic Center Boulevard, Philadelphia, PA 19104, USA; [c] Division of Transplantation, Department of Surgery, University of Pennsylvania Perelman School of Medicine, 3400 Spruce Street, Philadelphia, PA 19104-4283, USA
* Corresponding author. Division of Transplant Surgery, Department of Surgery, University of Wisconsin Hospital and Clinics, 600 Highland Avenue, Clinical Science Cntr-H4/772, Madison, WI 53792.
E-mail address: rrredfield@wisc.edu

or continuous subcutaneous insulin infusion pumps for survival. However, owing to the pharmacokinetic and pharmacodynamic limitations of subcutaneous insulin delivery, most patients living today in the United States with T1DM cannot achieve the degree of glycemic control (hemoglobin $A_{1c} < 7\%$) recommended by the American Diabetes Association.[1] Thus, with the discovery of insulin in 1922, T1DM has changed from a fatal disease to a chronic disease with serious secondary complications resulting from hyperglycemia that manifest many years after disease onset, including retinopathy, nephropathy, neuropathy, and cardiovascular disease.

Pancreas transplantation is a proven therapeutic treatment option for adults with insulin-dependent diabetes and is superior to intensive insulin therapy with regard to the efficacy of achieving normoglycemia and control of diabetic secondary complications. Despite improving outcomes for patient and graft survival, the rate of pancreas transplants performed in the United States has steadily decreased since the early 2000s (**Fig. 1**). The exact reasons for this decline are not fully understood, but potentially include changes in referral patterns, improvements in insulin delivery technologies resulting in delayed progression to advanced diabetic nephropathy, and changes in patient demographics shifting toward more obesity affecting patients with T1DM. A recent decrease in donor organ quality is also likely a contributing factor, because only approximately 15% of US deceased donors in 2013 donated a pancreas for transplantation. This is not a surprising trend, given that the US donor population is becoming increasingly aged, obese, and diabetic, all factors that adversely affect pancreatic graft functional outcomes. Despite these adverse trends, overall short-term technical success rates of pancreas transplantation have improved in recent years.

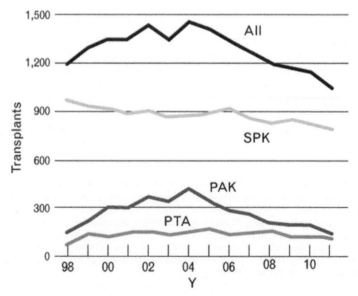

Fig. 1. Decreases in pancreatic transplant volume. Although still the most frequent of all forms of pancreas transplantation, SPK volumes have decreased since the late 1990s in the United States. PAK, pancreas after kidney; PTA, pancreas transplant alone; SPK, simultaneous kidney pancreas. (*From* Kandaswamy R, Stock PG, Skeans MA, et al. OPTN/SRTR 2011 annual data report: pancreas. Am J Transplant 2013;13(Suppl 1):47; with permission.)

CATEGORIES OF PANCREAS TRANSPLANTATION: SIMULTANEOUS PANCREAS AND KIDNEY TRANSPLANTATION, PANCREAS AFTER KIDNEY TRANSPLANTATION, AND PANCREAS TRANSPLANTATION ALONE: BROAD INDICATIONS

Simultaneous pancreas and kidney transplantations (SPK) constitute the majority of pancreas transplants performed in the United States, and account for approximately 70% of all pancreas transplants performed (see **Fig. 1**). An SPK, where the pancreas and kidney are recovered from the same donor and transplanted in the same operation to a single recipient, is indicated in adult patients with insulin-dependent diabetes and chronic renal failure of any cause. Although most candidates have kidney disease that is presumed owing to diabetes, in the occasional patient there are other or multifactorial causes. The addition of a pancreas at the time of kidney transplantation can normalize glucose control, providing immediate amelioration from hypoglycemia and metabolic instability and long-term stabilization and sometimes improvement of secondary diabetic complications. The uremic patient with diabetes is an excellent candidate for an SPK transplantation because the immunosuppressive medications that are needed are similar to those for a kidney transplant alone and they are often able to receive a high-quality deceased donor kidney with a shorter waiting time than if they were waiting for a deceased donor kidney transplant alone. As long as the cardiac and surgical risks of the dual operation are considered acceptable, the benefits of adding a pancreas transplant to ameliorate diabetes can extend to prolonging survival of the transplanted kidney that is protected by the pancreas from the development of recurrent diabetic nephropathy.[2]

The second most frequent category in which pancreas transplantation is performed is pancreas after kidney transplantation (PAK). A PAK can be offered to patients with T1DM who have received a previous kidney transplant from either a living or deceased donor or had a prior SPK and suffered loss of the pancreas allograft. This group accounts for approximately 20% of patients undergoing pancreas transplantations in the United States (see **Fig. 1**). An important consideration for this patient population is that of surgical risk and the state of their kidney allograft function, because other risks such as cardiac and immunosuppressive medication-related complications should be low when the patient has already demonstrated absence of cardiac events after the kidney transplant procedure and has tolerated the posttransplant medication regimen.

Pancreas transplantation alone (PTA) is indicated in selected patients with T1DM and normal native kidney function, and makes up the smallest percentage of pancreas transplants performed, roughly 10% (see **Fig. 1**). In this situation the key consideration, in addition to surgical risk, is an assessment of the risk of immunosuppression, and to determine if that risk is outweighed by the risk of diabetes treated with intensive insulin therapy. For these patients, the risk-versus-benefit calculation typically favors PTA in patients who are good surgical candidates with low cardiac risk profiles and who are unaware of impending hypoglycemia owing to loss of counterregulatory mechanisms and hypoglycemia-associated autonomic failure.[3] Various studies have estimated the frequency of hypoglycemia unawareness to be between 15% and 25% of patients.[4] These patients may have frequent and undetectable hypoglycemic episodes that can result in loss of consciousness and life-threatening accidents without warning. More subtly, but just as concerning for some patients, is the fact that frequent unanticipated hypoglycemia can affect employment, familial obligations such as child rearing, and the ability to keep a driver's license, as well as creating a constant state of fear in the patient and their caregivers. Clinical practice recommendations are available to guide assessment and management for the treatment of T1DM complications by such problematic hypoglycemia, including the consideration of pancreas, or where available outside the United States, isolated islet transplantation.[5] In other patients, a less common indication for PTA is severely labile glycemia that may be associated with frequent emergency room visits for diabetic ketoacidosis despite compliant behavior.

EXPANDING INDICATIONS FOR PANCREAS TRANSPLANTATION

Historically, pancreas transplantation has generally been considered suitable only for insulin-dependent T1DM patients, classically lean, ketosis prone, unable to produce insulin because of autoimmune β-cell destruction, with C-peptide levels that are extremely low or undetectable. This compares with T2DM patients, classically obese, insulin resistant, with inappropriately "normal" to elevated C-peptide levels. However, this binary understanding of diabetes fails to capture the clinical heterogeneity observed in clinical practice. There are retrospective data that support the application of pancreas transplantation to insulin-dependent patients with T2DM that are carefully selected by body mass index (BMI) and insulin requirement criteria to avoid significant insulin resistance and can become normoglycemic after pancreas transplantation. Because such patients less commonly experience the problematic hypoglycemia and related glycemic lability more often present in long-standing T1DM, non-T1DM account for 8% to 10% of SPK transplants performed in the United States and only 5% and 1% of PAK and PTA transplants are performed in this setting.[6]

Nevertheless, because of the rapidly increasing numbers of uremic T2DM patients, and the perceived concern that T2DM patients would overwhelm the current national transplant system, the United Network for Organ Sharing (UNOS) issued regulations that define eligibility criteria for patients with measurable C-peptide as a surrogate for T2DM. In essence, these regulations impose limits on the number of T2DM patients that will receive SPK transplants by restricting eligibility to those patients with a C-peptide of greater than 2 ng/mL and a BMI of less than 28 kg/m^2. UNOS policy mandates a 6-month review process with allowance for reduction (or increase) in the BMI eligibility threshold by plus or minus 2 kg/m^2 depending on the makeup and size of the waiting list.

Current data suggest that the outcomes are comparable between non-T1DM recipients and T1DM recipients.[7–10] Although in some series patient survival after SPK transplantation was worse in non-T1DM recipients compared with T1DM recipients, when adjusting for risk factors such as age, obesity, and African American ethnicity, outcomes were not inferior.[9,10] In addition, overall patient survival in the T2DM SPK patients was superior to those patients undergoing kidney transplantation alone.[8] Thus, in the appropriately selected T2DM patient, pancreas transplantation can be a valuable treatment option.[7,11,12]

Additional indications exist for pancreas transplantation in the setting of benign pancreatic disease.[13] These indications include other forms of diabetes as seen after pancreatectomy, performed either for chronic pancreatitis, pancreatic neoplasms (ie, intraductal papillary mucinous neoplasms), trauma, and various pediatric genetic abnormalities, and separately, in patients with cystic fibrosis who develop both pancreatic exocrine and endocrine insufficiency. In these postpancreatectomy and cystic fibrosis patients, there is the added benefit of restoring exocrine function with an enterically drained pancreas graft.[14,15]

An additional treatment approach for adult and pediatric patients with chronic pancreatitis, patients with benign pancreatic tumors, and traumatic pancreatic injury is that of total pancreatectomy and islet autotransplantation (TPIAT).[16–18] TPIAT has been associated with 70% to 80% resolution of pain rates and with significant insulin independence rates.[19] The success of insulin independence often depends on the severity of disease and whether the patient has had prior pancreatic surgery. If referred early before the destruction of native islets, or before attempted surgical drainage procedures, TPIAT can yield sufficient islets to achieve glycemic control with little or no exogenous insulin requirement.[17,18,20,21] In contrast with TPIAT, a subsequent pancreas transplant has the disadvantage of requiring lifelong immunosuppression, but the advantage of not only curing endocrine but also exocrine insufficiency. Both transplant options, if successful, can improve the recipient's quality of life.[22] Thus, for patients undergoing total pancreatectomy for nonmalignant disease, the standard of care is becoming TPIAT or subsequent pancreas transplantation.[16,22]

PRETRANSPLANT EVALUATION
Age and Body Mass Index

Many centers are reluctant to perform a pancreas transplant in patients older than 50 years of age and according to the International Pancreas Transplant Registry, only approximately 2% of pancreas transplants are performed in patients older than 60 years of age.[23] Historical data suggested that pancreas transplantation was associated with greater morbidity and mortality when recipients were over 45 years of age.[7] In the context of improved outcomes and the diabetes mellitus population living longer, older patients are now being listed for pancreas transplantation.[24]

Siskind and colleagues[25] published in 2014 a study of age-stratified pancreas transplantation outcomes using the UNOS/Scientific Registry of Transplant Recipients (SRTR) database. The investigators showed, not unexpectedly, that older patients (age 50–59) had shorter patient survival compared with younger patients. However, upon evaluation of death-censored graft survival, the authors observed minimal difference between various age groups.[25] There are few published data on the outcomes of pancreas transplantation in patients greater than 60 years of age, but many of the larger centers are now considering older patients to be potentially eligible as long as the patient has a favorable cardiovascular risk profile and does not have additional comorbidities.

The question of optimal BMI is also a sparsely studied topic. From historical, retrospective, single-center data, obesity has been considered a risk factor for reduced kidney and pancreas graft survival in SPK transplantation for many years.[26] Bedat and colleagues[27] recently addressed the impact of recipient BMI on pancreas transplant outcomes in all 3 pancreas transplant categories using the UNOS/SRTR registry in a comprehensive fashion. The authors demonstrate that (1) overweight ($25 \text{ kg/m}^2 < \text{BMI} < 29.9 \text{ kg/m}^2$) and obesity (BMI $\geq 30.0 \text{ kg/m}^2$) are associated with a moderate increase in early mortality, (2) overweight and obesity are associated with a moderate increased early pancreas graft loss, (3) obesity, but not overweight, is associated with poorer long-term graft survival, and (4) underweight (BMI $<18.5 \text{ kg/m}^2$) is associated with poorer long-term patient survival. Although the mechanisms underlying these findings are not understood clearly at this time, recipient BMI is a risk factor for recurrent diabetes developing after pancreas transplantation, and current evidence supports the best glycemic control outcomes with a pretransplant BMI of less than 28 kg/m^2 and prevention of posttransplant weight gain.[28,29] These are important data to consider in light of the increasing BMI of the diabetic population across the United States, and highlight the critical role for both pretransplant and posttransplant medical nutrition and behavioral modification treatment to achieve and maintain healthy body weight.

Cardiac Evaluation

Cardiovascular disease is the most important comorbidity in patients with diabetes, especially those with diabetic nephropathy. Because of the neuropathy associated with diabetes, patients are often asymptomatic, and the prevalence of significant coronary artery disease in patients with uremic diabetes is estimated to be approximately 40% to 60%. As such, screening studies to detect significant and treatable coronary artery disease is important in the evaluation for pancreas transplant candidacy. In our experience, noninvasive stress test screening misses approximately 50% of pancreas transplant patients who have significant coronary artery disease. Thus, with a high false-negative rate of noninvasive stress tests, high prevalence, and asymptomatic presentation, there is a "perfect storm" for the development of major cardiac events in the perioperative period. Risk factors such as age, duration of dialysis, duration of diabetes, and smoking and family history should be assessed but are not sufficiently predictive, and standard cardiac risk assessment tools have not been validated widely in this population. Hence, we have adopted an aggressive policy of coronary angiography in nearly all dialysis patients and the majority of nonuremic patients. In the pre-uremic patient, however, this can still present a diagnostic challenge because of the risk of iodinated contrast precipitating dialysis. Fortunately, techniques for coronary angiography have improved significantly and with the avoidance of ventriculograms such that the contrast dye load and consequently the nephrotoxic risk has been reduced considerably. We feel that the benefit of adequately screening these patients outweighs the risk of converting these patients to dialysis dependence and should not serve as an absolute justification to hold off on coronary angiography. Patients with coronary lesions amenable to angioplasty/stenting or bypass grafting should be treated, reevaluated, and then reconsidered for transplantation. The goal of revascularization is to diminish the perioperative risk of significant myocardial ischemia and cardiac events and to prolong the duration of life after transplantation. Patients who have experienced long waiting periods before pancreas transplantation should have their cardiac status reassessed at regular intervals.

Assessment of Peripheral Vascular Disease

Given the high rate of peripheral vascular disease present in the pancreas transplant population it is important to assess the adequacy of the iliac vessels before transplantation. A nonintravenous contrast computed tomography (CT) scan of the abdomen and pelvis is the best option for assessing target vessels, even at times when the clinical examination shows good femoral pulses. A noncontrast CT scan can easily detect iliac artery calcifications as well as aid in operative planning.

Additionally, diabetic patients are at risk for amputation of the lower extremity. These problems typically begin with a foot ulcer associated with advanced neuropathy and/or tibioperoneal vascular disease. Significant distal vascular disease or amputation of the lower extremities is not, however, an absolute contraindication to transplantation.

Assessment of Insulin Requirements, C-peptide, and Autoimmunity

Daily insulin requirements and serum fasting C-peptide levels are assessed to determine the type of diabetes present, the degree of insulin resistance, and so whether the patient will benefit from pancreas transplantation. Patients with high insulin requirements (eg, >1.0 U/kg per day) and high fasting C-peptide levels (eg, >4.0 ng/mL) probably have significant insulin resistance and may not be rendered insulin independent with a pancreas transplant. As an exception, patients who are on peritoneal dialysis may have large insulin requirements owing to the use of dextrose-containing dialysate; this should be taken into consideration when such patients are assessed for transplantation because their insulin requirement will likely decrease when peritoneal dialysis is discontinued after transplantation.

Few studies have examined criteria for pretransplant insulin requirements and C-peptide, which is challenging owing to varying renal insulin and C-peptide clearance mechanisms in patients with stage 4 and 5 chronic kidney disease undergoing transplant evaluation. In addition to kidney function that affects C-peptide clearance, it is important to interpret the C-peptide level with consideration of a concomitantly measured serum glucose that affects C-peptide secretion, because the level may be suppressed in insulin-treated patients experiencing hypoglycemia at the time of collection. The UNOS pancreas allocation system dictates that candidates will have to meet the following criteria for pancreas listing: on insulin and C-peptide 2 ng/mL or less (presumably T1DM) or on insulin and C-peptide greater than 2 ng/mL and BMI less than 28 to 30 kg/m^2 (presumably T2DM).

Finally, for patients with T1DM, pretransplant assessment of autoimmune markers (eg, antibodies against glutamic acid decarboxylase, insulinoma-associated antigen-2, zinc transporter-8, and insulin) should be considered to establish a baseline before possible pancreas transplantation. After transplantation, a new or increasing titer of a T1DM-specific autoantibody may indicate recurrent autoimmunity as a cause for pancreas graft dysfunction and aid in the evaluation of any new-onset hyperglycemia.[30,31]

Assessment of Problematic Hypoglycemia

Complications of long-standing T1DM, including the development of defective glucose counterregulation and hypoglycemic unawareness, related excessive glycemic lability, and frequent and severe hypoglycemia episodes, may increase the urgency for pancreas transplantation.[32] The most common tool used to assess hypoglycemia awareness is the Clarke Hypoglycemia Symptom Questionnaire. The Clarke method[33] comprises 8 questions characterizing the patient's exposure to episodes of moderate and severe hypoglycemia. It also examines the glycemic threshold for, and symptomatic responses to, hypoglycemia. A score of 4 or greater implies impaired awareness of hypoglycemia, and should be part of the evaluation of all T1DM patients considering pancreas transplantation.[5,34] Other more complicated, but more quantitative scoring systems include the Lability Index and the HYPO Score.[34,35]

Kidney Function

UNOS requires SPK candidates to meet criteria for kidney transplant listing (estimate glomerular filtration rate [eGFR]$\leq$ 20 mL/min or dialysis dependence). For both PAK and PTA candidates, the adequacy of kidney function should be assessed. Unfortunately, some patients being evaluated for PTA may have renal function that is too marginal for PTA but also not advanced enough to be eligible for SPK.[5] In these circumstances, where a PTA candidate has marginal renal function, a trial of tacrolimus therapy can be used to predict the effect of calcineurin inhibitor therapy on postoperative native kidney function. If native kidney functional reserve is deemed insufficient, then the patient is best served by waiting for kidney function to further deteriorate to an eGFR of 20 mL/min or less. The precise eGFR threshold for eligibility for PTA has not been determined, but many experienced centers recommend PTA candidates have an eGFR of greater than 70 to 80 mL/min and allow for microalbuminuria but not macroalbuminuria. The goal is to avoid PTA in patients with vulnerable kidney function owing to early underlying diabetic nephropathy. Because PAK patients are already on CNIs, the threshold for satisfactory kidney function is much lower and patients can be successfully transplanted with a PAK with an eGFR of approximately 40 to 50 mL/min with an expectation of little change in eGFR after pancreas transplantation.

Assessment of Autonomic Neuropathy

Autonomic neuropathy is prevalent in diabetic patients and may manifest as neurogenic bladder dysfunction, gastropathy, and/or orthostatic hypotension. Neurogenic bladder dysfunction is important to consider, especially in patients receiving a bladder-drained pancreas or an SPK transplant. A patient who is unable to empty the bladder completely or who cannot sense a full bladder may predispose the patient to urine reflux and high postvoid residuals. In the long term, these problems may adversely affect renal allograft function, increase the incidence of urinary tract infections, or lead to graft pancreatitis. Impaired gastric emptying is an important consideration with significant implications in the posttransplant period. Patients with severe gastroparesis may have difficulty tolerating oral immunosuppressive medications, predisposing the patient to subtherapeutic levels and graft rejection.

Assessment of Retinopathy

Diabetic retinopathy is a common finding in patients with diabetes and microangiopathy. Although blindness is not an absolute contraindication to transplantation, proper social support should be confirmed to ensure adequate support to help with travel and immunosuppressive medications in the patient with significant vision loss. Annual ophthalmologic examinations are recommended pretransplantation and posttransplantation. Acute normalization of glycemia has been associated with transient worsening of retinopathy, and so stability of retinopathy and provision of any indicated treatment should be ensured before pancreas transplantation.

Screen for Availability of Living Donors

Pursuing a living donor kidney (LDK) transplant before pancreas transplantation (ie, pancreas after LDK) is a viable alternative option for uremic T1DM patients instead of an SPK. The benefits of an LDK versus deceased donor SPK have been discussed in many forums.[36–38] A reasonable strategy to transplant a kidney and pancreas graft as rapidly as possible in this population is as follows: (i) if the patient does not have an LD, then the best option is an SPK, (ii) if the patient has 1 or more LDs then workup these donors, (iii) if the LDs are HLA identical, proceed with the HLA-identical LDK transplant first followed by a PAK transplant because these kidney grafts have superior long-term survival, (iv) if the LD is a haplotype match or less, then consider an LDK first only if there is a long waiting time for SPK, because receiving an LDK can reduce excess waiting list mortality, and (v) if on the other hand there is a short waiting time for SPK, then it is recommended to proceed with SPK because this option achieves rapid correction of uremia and diabetes with a high-quality kidney and equal short-term and long-term kidney allograft survival to haplotype-matched LDKs. Although initially controversial, recent literature supports increased or equivalent survival in patients who receive a pancreas after LDK versus LDK transplant alone.[28,39] Additionally, some studies demonstrate improved eGFR in patients after pancreas after LDK versus LDK transplant alone up to 10 years after transplantation.[40–42]

DONOR SELECTION

The criteria to select an adequate pancreas donor are much more stringent than for kidney transplantation. The most important criteria are based on direct visualization of the pancreas by an experienced pancreas transplant surgeon. A judgment then can be made regarding the degree of fibrosis, adipose tissue infiltration into the parenchyma, trauma, and specific vascular anomalies. One can predict some of these features before sending a donor team by certain donor characteristics namely age, BMI, and history of diabetes and alcohol abuse. Even when these donor characteristics are favorable, the pancreas may still be found to not be suitable for transplantation based on direct visualization. Acceptable deceased pancreas organ donors are typically between the ages of 5 and 55. The lower age limit is not based on perceived inadequate organ function but rather on whether the transplant is technically feasible given the small size of the splenic artery in a younger pancreas donor. Older pancreata have shown to be more prone to thrombosis, posttransplant pancreatitis, and decreased pancreas graft survival rates.[43] Donor BMI is also an important consideration. Obese donors (>30 kg/m^2) are frequently found not to be suitable pancreas donors. Obese patients often have a history of type 2 diabetes or the pancreas may be found to be unsuitable for transplantation because of a high degree of adipose infiltration of the pancreas, which does not preserve well, becomes necrotic, and is a potential nidus for infection. Many retrospective analyses have consistently identified donor age and BMI as the 2 most important factors that correlate with worse outcomes after pancreas transplantation.[44,45]

Donors with circulatory death pancreata can be transplanted successfully, as several studies have demonstrated.[46,47] The warm ischemia time, or time from extubation to asystole should ideally be less than 30 to 45 minutes. That donors with circulatory death kidneys are associated with greater rates of delayed kidney graft function in uremic SPK transplant recipients,[47,48] and that delayed kidney graft function in an SPK recipient is associated with higher rates of early pancreatic complications and graft loss, are also important considerations.[49]

To aid the transplant team in deciding on the quality of the potential donor pancreas, a pancreas donor risk index has been developed to inform organ acceptance decision making, which considers 10 common donor variables and 1 transplant variable (ischemia time) as factors affecting pancreas allograft survival.[50] Additionally, Finger and colleagues[44] generated a composite model to predict early technical failure of the pancreas allograft. They identified donor history of pancreatitis, donor age greater than 50, donor creatinine of 2.5 or greater, donor BMI 30 kg/m^2 or greater, and cold preservation time of greater than 20 hours as predictors of pancreas graft failure. The presence of 1 risk factor had little impact on the technical failure rate, but 2 or more conferred a significantly increased risk for technical failure. These findings highlight our belief that, to obtain good outcomes in pancreas transplantation, accepting more than 1 risk factor should be avoided. Incorporating these risk factors for technical failure along with the pancreas donor risk index, donor history, and direct visualization of the pancreas all must be taken into consideration when selecting donor pancreata for transplantation (**Fig. 2**).

Another important donor consideration is the static preservation solution. For abdominal organs, the 2 most commonly used preservative solutions in the United States are University of Wisconsin (UW) solution and histidine–tryptophan–ketoglutarate (HTK). In a retrospective UNOS/SRTR analysis, the use of HTK to preserve the pancreas graft increased the risk of pancreas graft loss (hazard ratio, 1.30; $P = .014$), especially in pancreas allografts with a cold ischemia time of 12 hours or longer (hazard ratio, 1.42; $P = .017$) compared with the use of UW solution.[51] This lesser survival with HTK preservation as compared with UW preservation was seen in both SPK transplants and PTA transplants. These results call into question the use of HTK for pancreas transplantation. Thus, currently in the United States the majority of abdominal organ recoveries are done with UW solution.

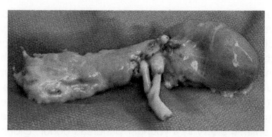

Fig. 2. Ideal pancreas for transplantation with arterial Y graft. (*From* Becker Y. Kidney and pancreas transplantation. In: Sabiston DC, Townsend CM, eds. Sabiston textbook of surgery: the biological basis of modern surgical practice. 19th edition. Philadelphia: Elsevier Saunders; 2012; with permission.)

RECIPIENT OPERATION

The evolution of pancreas transplantation has undergone significant modification since the first successful pancreas transplant was performed at the University of Minnesota in 1966. Although a detailed discussion on the technical aspects of pancreas transplantation is beyond the scope of this article, it is important to be aware of some general concepts. After procurement of the donor pancreas, the spleen is removed, a rim of donor duodenum is left attached to the head of the pancreas with oversewn ends to prevent a leak from the staple line, and the arterial supply of the pancreas is reconstructed with a Y-graft derived from the donor iliac artery bifurcation. Typically, the internal iliac artery is anastomosed to the splenic artery, and the external iliac artery is anastomosed to the stump of the superior mesenteric artery (see **Fig. 2**). The surgical techniques for implanting the pancreas are defined according to the mode of insulin venous delivery (systemic vs portal drainage) and the pancreatic exocrine drainage (enteric vs bladder drainage). Initially, management of the exocrine pancreas secretions was most commonly accomplished by bladder drainage, where the duodenum is anastomosed to the dome of the bladder (**Fig. 3**A). However, with the arrival of better immunosuppression, which has allowed for the successful healing of an enteric anastomosis, the preferred duct management technique has become enteric drainage, where the donor duodenum is sewn to the proximal jejunum (see **Fig. 3**B).

Complications of a bladder-drained pancreas are not trivial and include significant metabolic acidosis from pancreatic bicarbonate loss, and dehydration from volume loss. Urologic complications include urinary tract infections, cystitis, hematuria, urethritis, urethral stricture, and urethral disruption from exposure of the urothelium to injurious pancreatic enzymes, and reflux pancreatitis related to neurogenic bladder dysfunction, such that the majority of bladder-drained patients have been converted to enteric drainage.[2] Some centers prefer bladder drainage only for PTA to monitor for rejection (by measuring urine amylase), in contrast with an SPK where a biopsy of the simultaneously transplanted kidney can establish rejection.[52] We have not adopted this strategy for 2 reasons primarily: (1) we find pancreas biopsy to be more precise for rejection diagnosis and (2) the risks of urologic complications of bladder-drained grafts outweigh the risk of pancreas biopsy complications.

Some interest has been generated in the past about portal venous drainage as being a more physiologically relevant method for insulin delivery (**Fig. 4**). Although some reports of hyperinsulinism have been published with systemic venous drainage[53] the extra time and surgical risk associated with establishing portal venous drainage does

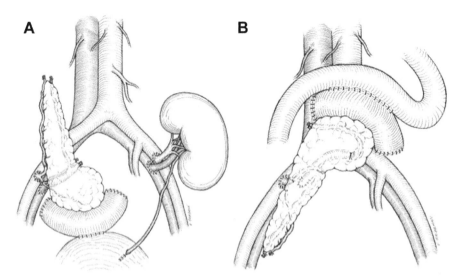

Fig. 3. Whole-organ pancreas transplantation with systemic venous drainage. The pancreas is placed in the right side of the pelvis with anastomosis of the donor portal vein to the recipient iliac vein for venous drainage. The donor iliac artery Y-graft is sewn to the recipient iliac artery for arterial inflow to the graft. Kidney transplantation can be performed simultaneously with the left-sided iliac vessels. (*A*) The donor duodenum is oriented inferiorly to allow anastomosis to the recipient bladder (shown) or to the recipient small intestine (not shown) for pancreatic exocrine drainage. (*B*) Alternatively, the donor duodenum is oriented superiorly to allow anastomosis to the recipient small intestine for pancreatic exocrine drainage. (*From* Desai NM, Markmann JF. Transplantation of the pancreas. In: Cameron JL, Cameron, AM. Current surgical therapy. 11th edition. Philadelphia: Elsevier Saunders; 2013; with permission.)

not justify the widespread use of this technique, especially given the equivalent long-term functional outcomes.[54]

Although there still exists diversity in operative techniques across the world, the majority of experienced centers elect to perform the pancreas transplantation with systemic venous drainage and enteric exocrine drainage (see **Fig. 3**B). Typically, the operation is performed by a midline laparotomy incision without the routine use of intravenous heparin and patients rarely require a stay in the intensive care unit. We do not routinely place a nasogastric tube allowing for quicker diet advancement and a shorter duration of stay.[55] Currently, our average duration of stay after pancreas transplantation is approximately 7 days.

IMMUNOSUPPRESSION

Immunosuppressive protocols for pancreas transplantation follow patterns similar to other solid organ transplants. Pancreas transplant recipients are believed to require higher levels of immunosuppression, possibly related to the increased immunogenicity of the composite pancreaticoduodenal graft, and/or underlying autoimmune status of the recipient. Unfortunately, given the low-volume nature of pancreas transplantation, the evidence for advantages or disadvantages of specific immunosuppressive regimens is quite limited. Currently, most centers use induction therapy with a T-cell–depleting antibody, such as antithymocyte globulin or alemtuzumab,[6,56] or less often an interleukin-2 receptor blocking antibody such as basiliximab.[56,57] For

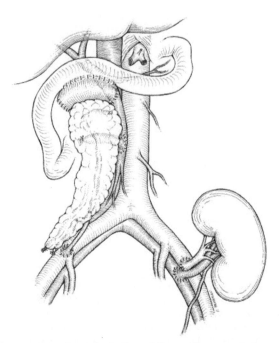

Fig. 4. Whole-organ pancreas transplantation with portal venous drainage. The pancreas is placed in the mid abdomen with anastomosis of the donor portal vein to the major branch of the recipient superior mesenteric vein for venous drainage. The donor iliac artery Y-graft is sewn to the recipient iliac artery for arterial inflow to the graft. The donor duodenum is oriented in the superior direction for anastomosis to the recipient small intestine. Kidney transplantation can be performed simultaneously with either the left (shown) or right iliac vessels. (*From* Desai NM, Markmann JF. Transplantation of the pancreas. In: Cameron JL, Cameron, AM. Current surgical therapy. 11th edition. Philadelphia: Elsevier Saunders; 2013; with permission.)

maintenance therapy, more than 80% of pancreas transplant recipients receive the calcineurin inhibitor tacrolimus and the purine synthesis inhibitor mycophenolate mofetil.[6,56] Glucocorticoids are used in more than 60% of recipients. Glucocorticoid use has increased slightly in recent years, despite interest and positive results of small steroid avoidance trials.[6] Most patients remain on physiologic doses of glucocorticoids, the equivalent of 5 mg of prednisone daily, whereas those patients who are not on steroids typically went through early steroid withdrawal protocols. Additionally, very few current immunosuppressive protocols for SPK involve mammalian target of rapamycin inhibitors. The standard regimen of antibody induction and maintenance with tacrolimus, mycophenolate mofetil, with or without glucocorticoids has ushered in an era of routine success in pancreas transplantation, with 1-year pancreas allograft survival near or exceeding 90%.[6,58] In addition to providing protection against alloimmune rejection and recurrent autoimmunity, modern dosing of tacrolimus-based regimens is not toxic to islet β-cells, as evidenced by normal β-cell secretory capacity in pancreas transplant recipients.[59]

SURGICAL COMPLICATIONS AND PANCREAS REJECTION

The most common complications in enterically drained transplants in the early postoperative period are provided in **Box 1**. These complications, although infrequent,

Box 1
Potential early complications of pancreatic transplantation
Thrombosis
Arterial
Venous
Hemorrhage
Pancreatic graft
Vascular anastomosis
Infection
Bacterial or fungal
Peripancreatic fluid
Superficial wound
Urinary tract
Metabolic
Acidosis
Hyperkalemia, hypokalemia, hypocalcemia, and hypomagnesemia
Dehydration
Gastrointestinal
Anastomotic leak (enteric-drained graft)
Mechanical obstruction
Urologic
Hematuria
Bladder anastomotic leak (bladder-drained graft)
Urethral injury/stenosis

typically present within the initial hospital course or shortly thereafter (within the first month). However, they can also present after discharge and the patient should be referred back to the transplant center to treat these complications appropriately. The likelihood of acute surgical complications decreases with time, but other complications, including rejection, become more prevalent during this later timeframe (**Fig. 5**).

Rejection is most often heralded by an increase in pancreatic enzymes, with lipase being more sensitive than amylase; most patients are asymptomatic on presentation. When asymptomatic, the source of the increased enzymes is often from the insensate transplanted pancreas, but unfortunately it is not a specific marker for rejection. Symptomatic increases in pancreatic enzymes can point to either transplant or native gland disease. Because signs and symptoms of pancreatic graft dysfunction can arise from multiple causes in the setting of an enterically drained pancreas graft, it is helpful to consider both the timing of presentation and the differential diagnosis when evaluating these patients (see **Fig. 5**).

An algorithm that these authors use in practice for the diagnosis and management of patients with increased pancreatic enzymes is shown in **Fig. 6**. In our practice, the initial approach to the patient with elevated enzymes is history and physical, fasting C-peptide, hemoglobin A_{1c}, donor-specific antibodies, and an imaging study,

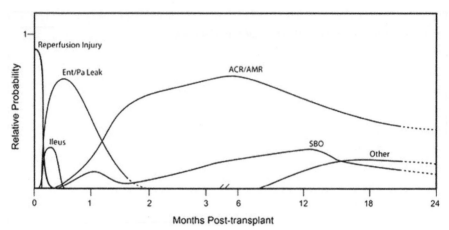

Fig. 5. Temporal relationship of elevated pancreas enzymes to etiology. Surgical complications typically present early in the postoperative course, whereas rejection most commonly presents later. "Other" includes possible causes, such as transplant pancreatic duct stricture, native pancreatitis, intraductal papillary mucinous neoplasms or cancer in pancreas transplant or native pancreas, and penetrating ulcer. Of note, although complete graft thrombosis can present as increased pancreatic enzymes, in our experience, this is a very uncommon presentation, and when most grafts thrombose, very limited increases in enzymes are seen if at all. Relative probability on the y-axis does not represent the overall probability or incidence of this complication; instead, it strives to convey the relative probability that these diagnoses are associated with elevated pancreatic enzymes. ACR, acute cellular rejection; Ent/Pa Leak, enteric or pancreatic leak; SBO, small bowel obstruction. (*From* Redfield RR, Kaufman DB, Odorico JS. Diagnosis and treatment of pancreas rejection. Curr Transplant Rep 2015;2:169; with permission.)

preferably CT scan of the abdomen and pelvis with intravenous and oral contrast to evaluate for postoperative complications or intraabdominal infection before performing a pancreas allograft biopsy (see **Fig. 6**).

Pancreas allograft biopsies are typically performed for specific indications, such as elevated pancreatic enzymes, fever of unknown origin, or mild hyperglycemia. Percutaneous biopsies are most commonly done using real-time ultrasound or CT fluoroscopy guidance. With experience biopsies can be perform with a very low risks.[60] We have performed well over 400 percutaneous biopsies with a very low complication rate and no graft losses. Two patients required reoperation: one for bleeding and one for control of pancreatic ascites, which ultimately resolved, and both patients currently still retain excellent graft function. We prefer ultrasound-guided biopsy with an 18-gauge automatic biopsy device. Our trajectory for biopsy is ideally toward the tail, avoiding the splenic artery and vein. Because of the nest of vessels and larger duct in the head region, we prefer to biopsy the body/tail of the graft aiming either transversely or preferably longitudinally with respect to the axis of the pancreas.

Standardized guidelines for the diagnosis of pancreas rejection focusing on acute cellular rejection were published by the Banff working group in 2007[61] and in response to reports in the literature documenting pancreas antibody-mediated rejection,[62,63] the Banff guidelines were updated in 2011 to include comprehensive guidelines for diagnosis of acute and chronic antibody-mediated rejection of the pancreas.[64]

There are limited data in the literature on which to base a practice strategy for the treatment of pancreas rejection. In this context, treatment strategies have been extrapolated from the kidney transplant literature. Our pancreas rejection treatment

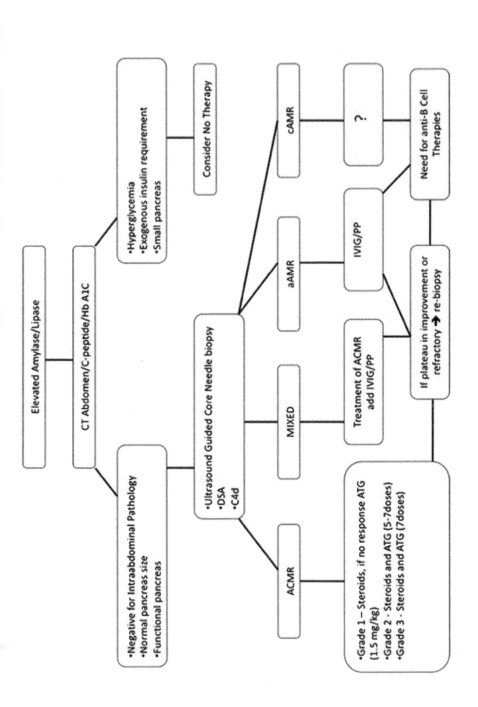

algorithm is shown in **Fig. 6**. Overall, key points of this treatment algorithm are as follows:

1. Ensure that the pancreas is still functioning and therefore worthy of salvage;
2. Obtain tissue diagnosis to evaluate the grade of rejection and the relative contribution of acute cellular rejection and antibody-mediated rejection to graft dysfunction;
3. Treat acute cellular rejection aggressively as a first and primary strategy;
4. Sequentially escalate therapy as data become available and/or if there is no improvement in enzymes with acute cellular rejection–directed treatment; and
5. If there is doubt as to the cause of ongoing enzyme elevation or hyperglycemia, it is valuable to consider rebiopsy.

Although we acknowledge that the current understanding of pancreas rejection and treatment are still evolving and more study is warranted, we believe this approach is a reasonable management protocol that has resulted in very low recurrence rates and excellent postrejection graft survival.[65]

IMPROVING OUTCOMES, BENEFIT TO QUALITY OF LIFE, AND END-ORGAN COMPLICATIONS

The half-life for an SPK pancreatic graft has steadily increased to more than 14 years currently (**Fig. 7**).[6] This is likely the result of a variety of factors, including improved operative technique, immunosuppression, donor and recipient selection, and graft surveillance, with greater reliance on pancreas biopsy.[66] The rates of patient survival are approximately 97% at 1 year and 92% at 3 years after SPK transplantation. Similar patient survival rates are reported for PAK and PTA recipients. Graft survival is variable, depending on the type of pancreas transplant performed (**Fig. 8**). According to recent SRTR data, 1- and 3-year pancreas graft survival rates for SPK are 89% and 80%, respectively. For PAK and PTA recipients, 1- and 3-year pancreas graft survival rates are 84% and 66% and 80% and 60%, respectively. SPK transplant pancreas graft survival continues to be higher than that for solitary pancreas grafts and graft survival and insulin independence rates for all categories continue to improve. Additionally, the mortality benefit of pancreas transplantation is well-documented. The mortality among diabetics is greatly reduced by SPK transplantation compared with the waiting list; however, it is less so for solitary pancreas transplants.[2,67]

The remarkable advances in transplantation technology and progressive improvements in long-term graft survival in the current era promise to provide significant patient survival and quality-of-life benefits beyond those documented already in the literature. That said, historical literature and personal experience indicate the effects of restoring normoglycemia and insulin independence on patient's quality of life cannot be understated. Studies have demonstrated that patients rate their lives better after pancreas transplantation than before mainly owing to freedom from frequent blood glucose monitoring, insulin therapy, and hypoglycemia.[68,69] Normalization of glycemic control may benefit the long-term retinal, nephrologic, neurologic, and macrovascular complications of diabetes.[70–73] Successful pancreas transplantation has

◀───────────────────────────

Fig. 6. The University of Wisconsin Diagnosis and Treatment Algorithm. aAMR, acute antibody-mediated rejection; ACMR, acute cell-mediated rejection; ATG, antithymocyte globulin; cAMR, chronic antibody-mediated rejection; CT, computed tomography; DSA, donor-specific antibody; IVIG, intravenous immunoglobulin; PP, plasmapheresis. (*From* Redfield RR, McCune KR, Sollinger HW, et al. Pancreas allograft antibody mediated rejection: current concepts and future therapies. Trends Transplan 2014, in press; with permission.)

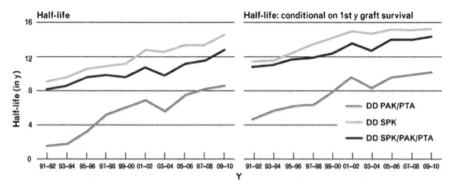

Fig. 7. Improving results of SPK transplantation in the United States. The half-life for an SPK is now approximately 14 years. DD, deceased donor; PAK, pancreas after kidney; PTA, pancreas transplant alone; SPK, simultaneous kidney pancreas. (*From* Kandaswamy R, Stock PG, Skeans MA, et al. OPTN/SRTR 2011 annual data report: pancreas. Am J Transplant 2013;13(Suppl 1):47; with permission.)

been shown to eventually reverse established lesions of diabetic nephropathy by 10 years posttransplant.[70] There is stabilization and, in some cases, improvement in peripheral and autonomic diabetic neuropathy.[71,74] With regard to the potential of pancreas transplantation to halt or reverse diabetic retinopathy, some studies have not shown a benefit, whereas others have shown evidence for halting or reversing proliferative retinopathy.[75–78] Although there is evidence to the benefit of normalizing glucose control long term on microangiopathy, it has been more difficult to demonstrate improvements in macrovascular disease, such as cardiovascular and peripheral vascular disease, and their sequelae such as myocardial infarction and amputations, although some studies have reported benefit.[72] The reports of studies evaluating the

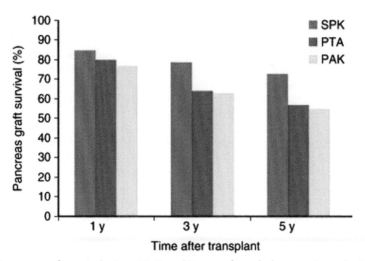

Fig. 8. Pancreas graft survival rates at 1, 3, and 5 years after whole organ transplantation by transplantation category. PAK, pancreas-after-kidney transplantation; PTA, pancreas transplantation alone; SPK, simultaneous kidney and pancreas transplantation. (*From* Desai NM, Markmann JF. Transplantation of the pancreas. In: Cameron JL, Cameron, AM. Current surgical therapy. 11th edition. Philadelphia: Elsevier Saunders; 2013; with permission.)

end-organ effects of pancreas transplantation need to be interpreted with caution because many are inadequately powered and lack appropriate control groups. Reexamining these questions in larger, controlled studies is certainly warranted.

SUMMARY

The field of pancreas transplantation has evolved from an experimental procedure in the 1980s to become a routine therapy in the modern era. With outcomes continuing to improve and the significant benefits on mortality, quality of life, and end-organ complications, indications for pancreas transplantation are expanding. Recent guidelines from the endocrinology community highlight the role of pancreas transplantation as a treatment for T1DM complicated by problematic hypoglycemia,[5] emphasizing consideration for patients beyond those with advanced kidney disease. Isolated islet transplantation is being developed in the United States (and is available in other countries) as a complementary alternative to pancreas transplantation that may use organs not suitable for solid organ transplantation and reach patients not candidates for or willing to accept the risks of the required surgery.[79] While islet and other emerging cell therapy and technologic approaches to the treatment of diabetes mature, pancreas transplantation remains the gold standard approach to β-cell replacement therapy against which novel interventions must prove their worth and distinction.[80,81]

REFERENCES

1. Miller KM, Foster NC, Beck RW, et al. Current state of type 1 diabetes treatment in the U.S.: updated data from the T1D Exchange clinic registry. Diabetes Care 2015;38:971.
2. Sollinger HW, Odorico JS, Becker YT, et al. One thousand simultaneous pancreas-kidney transplants at a single center with 22-year follow-up. Ann Surg 2009;250:618.
3. Cryer PE. Mechanisms of hypoglycemia-associated autonomic failure in diabetes. N Engl J Med 2013;369:362.
4. Frier BM, Fisher BM. Hypoglycaemia in clinical diabetes. 2nd edition. Chichester (England); Hoboken (NJ): John Wiley & Sons; 2007.
5. Choudhary P, Rickels MR, Senior PA, et al. Evidence-informed clinical practice recommendations for treatment of type 1 diabetes complicated by problematic hypoglycemia. Diabetes Care 2015;38:1016.
6. Israni AK, Skeans MA, Gustafson SK, et al. OPTN/SRTR 2012 annual data report: pancreas. Am J Transplant 2014;14(Suppl 1):45.
7. Orlando G, Stratta RJ, Light J. Pancreas transplantation for type 2 diabetes mellitus. Curr Opin Organ Transplant 2011;16:110.
8. Margreiter C, Resch T, Oberhuber R, et al. Combined pancreas-kidney transplantation for patients with end-stage nephropathy caused by type-2 diabetes mellitus. Transplantation 2013;95:1030.
9. Light J, Tucker M. Simultaneous pancreas kidney transplants in diabetic patients with end-stage renal disease: the 20-yr experience. Clin Transplant 2013;27: E256.
10. Sampaio MS, Kuo HT, Bunnapradist S. Outcomes of simultaneous pancreas-kidney transplantation in type 2 diabetic recipients. Clin J Am Soc Nephrol 2011;6:1198.
11. Sasaki TM, Gray RS, Ratner RE, et al. Successful long-term kidney-pancreas transplants in diabetic patients with high C-peptide levels. Transplantation 1998;65:1510.

12. Stratta RJ, Rogers J, Farney AC, et al. Pancreas transplantation in C-peptide positive patients: does "type" of diabetes really matter? J Am Coll Surg 2015; 220:716.
13. Mehrabi A, Golriz M, Adili-Aghdam F, et al. Expanding the indications of pancreas transplantation alone. Pancreas 2014;43:1190.
14. Fridell JA, Vianna R, Mangus RS, et al. Addition of a total pancreatectomy and pancreas transplantation in a liver transplant recipient with intraductal papillary mucinous neoplasm of the pancreas. Clin Transplant 2008;22:681.
15. Charpentier KP, Brentnall TA, Bronner MP, et al. A new indication for pancreas transplantation: high grade pancreatic dysplasia. Clin Transplant 2004;18:105.
16. Ris F, Niclauss N, Morel P, et al. Islet autotransplantation after extended pancreatectomy for focal benign disease of the pancreas. Transplantation 2011;91:895.
17. Balzano G, Maffi P, Nano R, et al. Extending indications for islet autotransplantation in pancreatic surgery. Ann Surg 2013;258:210.
18. Chinnakotla S, Bellin MD, Schwarzenberg SJ, et al. Total pancreatectomy and islet autotransplantation in children for chronic pancreatitis: indication, surgical techniques, postoperative management, and long-term outcomes. Ann Surg 2014;260:56.
19. Bramis K, Gordon-Weeks AN, Friend PJ, et al. Systematic review of total pancreatectomy and islet autotransplantation for chronic pancreatitis. Br J Surg 2012; 99:761.
20. Wang H, Desai KD, Dong H, et al. Prior surgery determines islet yield and insulin requirement in patients with chronic pancreatitis. Transplantation 2013;95:1051.
21. Kobayashi T, Manivel JC, Bellin MD, et al. Correlation of pancreatic histopathologic findings and islet yield in children with chronic pancreatitis undergoing total pancreatectomy and islet autotransplantation. Pancreas 2010;39:57.
22. Gruessner RW, Sutherland DE, Dunn DL, et al. Transplant options for patients undergoing total pancreatectomy for chronic pancreatitis. J Am Coll Surg 2004; 198:559.
23. Gruessner AC. 2011 update on pancreas transplantation: comprehensive trend analysis of 25,000 cases followed up over the course of twenty-four years at the International Pancreas Transplant Registry (IPTR). Rev Diabet Stud 2011;8:6.
24. Kandaswamy R, Skeans MA, Gustafson SK, et al. OPTN/SRTR 2013 annual data report: pancreas. Am J Transplant 2015;15(Suppl 2):1.
25. Siskind E, Maloney C, Akerman M, et al. An analysis of pancreas transplantation outcomes based on age groupings–an update of the UNOS database. Clin Transplant 2014;28:990.
26. Bumgardner GL, Henry ML, Elkhammas E, et al. Obesity as a risk factor after combined pancreas/kidney transplantation. Transplantation 1995;60:1426.
27. Bedat B, Niclauss N, Jannot AS, et al. Impact of recipient body mass index on short-term and long-term survival of pancreatic grafts. Transplantation 2015; 99:94.
28. Young BY, Gill J, Huang E, et al. Living donor kidney versus simultaneous pancreas-kidney transplant in type I diabetics: an analysis of the OPTN/UNOS database. Clin J Am Soc Nephrol 2009;4:845.
29. Neidlinger N, Singh N, Klein C, et al. Incidence of and risk factors for posttransplant diabetes mellitus after pancreas transplantation. Am J Transplant 2010;10:398.
30. Vendrame F, Pileggi A, Laughlin E, et al. Recurrence of type 1 diabetes after simultaneous pancreas-kidney transplantation, despite immunosuppression, is associated with autoantibodies and pathogenic autoreactive CD4 T-cells. Diabetes 2010;59:947.

31. Burke GW 3rd, Vendrame F, Pileggi A, et al. Recurrence of autoimmunity following pancreas transplantation. Curr Diab Rep 2011;11:413.

32. Rickels MR. Recovery of endocrine function after islet and pancreas transplantation. Curr Diab Rep 2012;12:587.

33. Clarke WL, Cox DJ, Gonder-Frederick LA, et al. Reduced awareness of hypoglycemia in adults with IDDM. A prospective study of hypoglycemic frequency and associated symptoms. Diabetes Care 1995;18:517.

34. Senior PA, Bellin MD, Alejandro R, et al. Consistency of quantitative scores of hypoglycemia severity and glycemic lability and comparison with continuous glucose monitoring system measures in long-standing type 1 diabetes. Diabetes Technol Ther 2015;17:235.

35. Ryan EA, Shandro T, Green K, et al. Assessment of the severity of hypoglycemia and glycemic lability in type 1 diabetic subjects undergoing islet transplantation. Diabetes 2004;53:955.

36. Wiseman AC. Pancreas transplant options for patients with type 1 diabetes mellitus and chronic kidney disease: simultaneous pancreas kidney or pancreas after kidney? Curr Opin Organ Transplant 2012;17:80.

37. Rayhill SC, D'Alessandro AM, Odorico JS, et al. Simultaneous pancreas-kidney transplantation and living related donor renal transplantation in patients with diabetes: is there a difference in survival? Ann Surg 2000;231:417.

38. Reese PP, Israni AK. Best option for transplant candidates with type 1 diabetes and a live kidney donor: a bird in the hand is worth two in the bush. Clin J Am Soc Nephrol 2009;4:700.

39. Sampaio MS, Poommipanit N, Cho YW, et al. Transplantation with pancreas after living donor kidney vs. living donor kidney alone in type 1 diabetes mellitus recipients. Clin Transplant 2010;24:812.

40. Morath C, Zeier M, Dohler B, et al. Transplantation of the type 1 diabetic patient: the long-term benefit of a functioning pancreas allograft. Clin J Am Soc Nephrol 2010;5:549.

41. Morath C, Zeier M, Dohler B, et al. Metabolic control improves long-term renal allograft and patient survival in type 1 diabetes. J Am Soc Nephrol 2008;19:1557.

42. Kleinclauss F, Fauda M, Sutherland DE, et al. Pancreas after living donor kidney transplants in diabetic patients: impact on long-term kidney graft function. Clin Transplant 2009;23:437.

43. Salvalaggio PR, Schnitzler MA, Abbott KC, et al. Patient and graft survival implications of simultaneous pancreas kidney transplantation from old donors. Am J Transplant 2007;7:1561.

44. Finger EB, Radosevich DM, Dunn TB, et al. A composite risk model for predicting technical failure in pancreas transplantation. Am J Transplant 2013;13:1840.

45. Humar A, Ramcharan T, Kandaswamy R, et al. Technical failures after pancreas transplants: why grafts fail and the risk factors–a multivariate analysis. Transplantation 2004;78:1188.

46. Salvalaggio PR, Davies DB, Fernandez LA, et al. Outcomes of pancreas transplantation in the United States using cardiac-death donors. Am J Transplant 2006;6:1059.

47. Fernandez LA, Di Carlo A, Odorico JS, et al. Simultaneous pancreas-kidney transplantation from donation after cardiac death: successful long-term outcomes. Ann Surg 2005;242:716.

48. Bellingham JM, Santhanakrishnan C, Neidlinger N, et al. Donation after cardiac death: a 29-year experience. Surgery 2011;150:692.

49. Muth B, Astor B, Kaufman D, et al. Delayed kidney graft function in SPK recipients is associated with poor long-term outcomes [abstract]. Am J Transplant 2013; 13(Suppl 5).
50. Axelrod DA, Sung RS, Meyer KH, et al. Systematic evaluation of pancreas allograft quality, outcomes and geographic variation in utilization. Am J Transplant 2010;10:837.
51. Stewart ZA, Cameron AM, Singer AL, et al. Histidine-tryptophan-ketoglutarate (HTK) is associated with reduced graft survival in pancreas transplantation. Am J Transplant 2009;9:217.
52. Burke GW, Gruessner R, Dunn DL, et al. Conversion of whole pancreaticoduodenal transplants from bladder to enteric drainage for metabolic acidosis or dysuria. Transplant Proc 1990;22:651.
53. Diem P, Abid M, Redmon JB, et al. Systemic venous drainage of pancreas allografts as independent cause of hyperinsulinemia in type I diabetic recipients. Diabetes 1990;39:534.
54. Gaber AO, Shokouh-Amiri MH, Hathaway DK, et al. Results of pancreas transplantation with portal venous and enteric drainage. Ann Surg 1995;221:613.
55. Barth RN, Becker YT, Odorico JS, et al. Nasogastric decompression is not necessary after simultaneous pancreas-kidney transplantation. Ann Surg 2008;247:350.
56. Mittal S, Johnson P, Friend P. Pancreas transplantation: solid organ and islet. Cold Spring Harb Perspect Med 2014;4:a015610.
57. Niederhaus SV, Kaufman DB, Odorico JS. Induction therapy in pancreas transplantation. Transpl Int 2013;26:704.
58. Ollinger R, Margreiter C, Bosmuller C, et al. Evolution of pancreas transplantation: long-term results and perspectives from a high-volume center. Ann Surg 2012; 256:780.
59. Rickels MR, Mueller R, Teff KL, et al. {beta}-Cell secretory capacity and demand in recipients of islet, pancreas, and kidney transplants. J Clin Endocrinol Metab 2010;95:1238.
60. Klassen DK, Weir MR, Cangro CB, et al. Pancreas allograft biopsy: safety of percutaneous biopsy-results of a large experience. Transplantation 2002; 73:553.
61. Drachenberg CB, Odorico J, Demetris AJ, et al. Banff schema for grading pancreas allograft rejection: working proposal by a multi-disciplinary international consensus panel. Am J Transplant 2008;8:1237.
62. Melcher ML, Olson JL, Baxter-Lowe LA, et al. Antibody-mediated rejection of a pancreas allograft. Am J Transplant 2006;6:423.
63. Torrealba JR, Samaniego M, Pascual J, et al. C4d-positive interacinar capillaries correlates with donor-specific antibody-mediated rejection in pancreas allografts. Transplantation 2008;86:1849.
64. Drachenberg CB, Torrealba JR, Nankivell BJ, et al. Guidelines for the diagnosis of antibody-mediated rejection in pancreas allografts-updated Banff grading schema. Am J Transplant 2011;11:1792.
65. Niederhaus SV, Leverson GE, Lorentzen DF, et al. Acute cellular and antibody-mediated rejection of the pancreas allograft: incidence, risk factors and outcomes. Am J Transplant 2013;13:2945.
66. Gruessner RW, Gruessner AC. The current state of pancreas transplantation. Nat Rev Endocrinol 2013;9:555.
67. Gruessner RW, Sutherland DE, Gruessner AC. Mortality assessment for pancreas transplants. Am J Transplant 2004;4:2018.

68. Nathan DM, Fogel H, Norman D, et al. Long-term metabolic and quality of life results with pancreatic/renal transplantation in insulin-dependent diabetes mellitus. Transplantation 1991;52:85.
69. Becker BN, Odorico JS, Becker YT, et al. Simultaneous pancreas-kidney and pancreas transplantation. J Am Soc Nephrol 2001;12:2517.
70. Fioretto P, Steffes MW, Sutherland DE, et al. Reversal of lesions of diabetic nephropathy after pancreas transplantation. N Engl J Med 1998;339:69.
71. Navarro X, Sutherland DE, Kennedy WR. Long-term effects of pancreatic transplantation on diabetic neuropathy. Ann Neurol 1997;42:727.
72. Jukema JW, Smets YF, van der Pijl JW, et al. Impact of simultaneous pancreas and kidney transplantation on progression of coronary atherosclerosis in patients with end-stage renal failure due to type 1 diabetes. Diabetes Care 2002;25:906.
73. Koznarova R, Saudek F, Sosna T, et al. Beneficial effect of pancreas and kidney transplantation on advanced diabetic retinopathy. Cell Transplant 2000;9:903.
74. Kennedy WR, Navarro X, Goetz FC, et al. Effects of pancreatic transplantation on diabetic neuropathy. N Engl J Med 1990;322:1031.
75. Ramsay RC, Goetz FC, Sutherland DE, et al. Progression of diabetic retinopathy after pancreas transplantation for insulin-dependent diabetes mellitus. N Engl J Med 1988;318:208.
76. Wang Q, Klein R, Moss SE, et al. The influence of combined kidney-pancreas transplantation on the progression of diabetic retinopathy. A case series. Ophthalmology 1994;101:1071.
77. Pearce IA, Ilango B, Sells RA, et al. Stabilisation of diabetic retinopathy following simultaneous pancreas and kidney transplant. Br J Ophthalmol 2000;84:736.
78. Konigsrainer A, Miller K, Steurer W, et al. Does pancreas transplantation influence the course of diabetic retinopathy? Diabetologia 1991;34(Suppl 1):S86.
79. Rickels MR, Liu C, Shlansky-Goldberg RD, et al. Improvement in beta-cell secretory capacity after human islet transplantation according to the CIT07 protocol. Diabetes 2013;62:2890.
80. Bartlett ST, MJ, Johnson P, et al. Report from the IPITA-TTS opinion leaders meeting on the future of beta cell replacement. Transplantation, in press.
81. Markmann JF, BS, Johnson P, et al. Executive summary of IPITA-TTS Opinion Leaders meeting on the future of beta cell replacement. Transplantation, in press.

Index

Note: Page numbers of article titles are in **boldface** type.

A

Adenocarcinoma
  high-risk populations for, **117–127**
  radiography for, 103–104
Age factors, pancreatic transplantation and, 149
Alemtuzumab, after pancreas transplantation, 155
Alliance for Clinical Trials in Oncology Intergroup F021101, 134–135
American College of Radiology, cystic neoplasm guidelines of, 74–78
American College of Surgeons, National Surgical Quality Improvement
    Program, 130–131
American Gastroenterology Association, cystic neoplasm guidelines of, 74–78
American Pancreatic Association, 137–138
The Americas Hepatopancreatobiliary Association, 134–135
Ampullary neoplasm, ERCP for, 56–57
Amylase, in cysts, 108
Antibiotics, for acute pancreatitis, 3–4
Antithymocyte globulin, after pancreas transplantation, 155
APC gene, in cancer, 121
Ascites, pancreatic duct leaks and, 55–56
Asian guidelines, for autoimmune pancreatitis, 31, 38
Ataxia-telangectasia, 121
ATM gene, in cancer, 118–119, 121
Autoimmune disease, pancreatic transplantation and, 150–151
Autoimmune pancreatitis, **19–43**
  clinical characteristics of, 30
  diagnosis of, 30–38
  ERCP for, 54–55
  history of, 29–30
  incidence of, 29
  treatment of, 38–40
Autonomic neuropathy, pancreatic transplantation and, 152
Axios stent, 17–18
Azathioprine, for autoimmune pancreatitis, 39–40

B

Balloon dilation, for pseudocyst drainage, 15, 19–20
Banff guidelines, for pancreas graft rejection, 158
Bevacizumab, for PNETs, 93
Biliary tract, decompression of, 56–57
Biomarkers, for cancer, 123–124

http://dx.doi.org/10.1016/S0889-8553(16)00013-3
0889-8553/16/$ – see front matter © 2016 Elsevier Inc. All rights reserved.

Moving?

Make sure your subscription moves with you!

To notify us of your new address, find your **Clinics Account Number** (located on your mailing label above your name), and contact customer service at:

Email: journalscustomerservice-usa@elsevier.com

800-654-2452 (subscribers in the U.S. & Canada)
314-447-8871 (subscribers outside of the U.S. & Canada)

Fax number: 314-447-8029

Elsevier Health Sciences Division
Subscription Customer Service
3251 Riverport Lane
Maryland Heights, MO 63043

*To ensure uninterrupted delivery of your subscription, please notify us at least 4 weeks in advance of move.

Printed and bound by CPI Group (UK) Ltd, Croydon, CR0 4YY

03/10/2024

01040486-0018